Medical Ethics - Navigating Complex Decisions in Contemporary Healthcare

Edited by Thomas F. Heston

Published in London, United Kingdom

Medical Ethics - Navigating Complex Decisions in Contemporary Healthcare
http://dx.doi.org/10.5772/intechopen.1008599
Edited by Thomas F. Heston

Contributors
Abigail Garba, Ana Mateus, Daisy Michelle Princeton, Daniela Oehring, David N. Durrheim, Franz Staudt, Gantulga Darambazar, Gelegjamts Delgersuren, Gülendam Hakverdioğlu Yönt, Ivo Laranjinha, Justin J. Gillette, Kudirat Busari, Michelle Lu, Noel Boyle, Omboosuren Bolorsaikhan, Omri-David Soffer, Pedro Ponce, Priya Hays, Sezer Kisa, Thomas F. Heston, Yvette Koepke

First published in London, United Kingdom, 2026 by IntechOpen
IntechOpen is the global imprint of INTECHOPEN LIMITED, registered in England and Wales, registration number: 11086078, 167-169 Great Portland Street, London, W1W 5PF, United Kingdom

For EU product safety concerns: IN TECH d.o.o., Prolaz Marije Krucifikse Kozulić 3, 51000 Rijeka, Croatia, info@intechopen.com or visit our website at intechopen.com.

British Library Cataloguing-in-Publication Data
A catalogue record for this book is available from the British Library

Medical Ethics - Navigating Complex Decisions in Contemporary Healthcare
Edited by Thomas F. Heston
p. cm.
Print ISBN 978-1-83635-902-9
Online ISBN 978-1-83635-901-2
eBook (PDF) ISBN 978-1-83635-903-6

Meet the editor

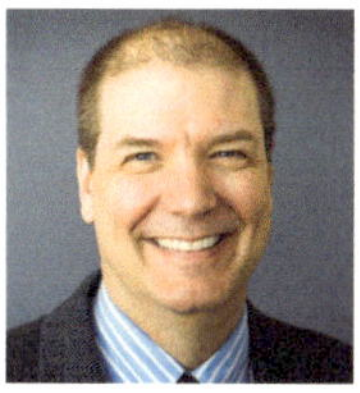

Thomas F. Heston, MD, MSc, serves as Clinical Assistant Professor in the Department of Family Medicine at the University of Washington and Clinical Associate Professor in the Department of Medical Education and Clinical Sciences at Washington State University. He completed medical school at Saint Louis University and earned his MSc in Cryptocurrency and Blockchain Technology from the University of Nicosia. His research focuses on the application and ethical implications of large language models in medical education and clinical practice. His work examines how artificial intelligence technologies transform clinical decision-making, reshape the physician-patient relationship, and challenge traditional frameworks for medical ethics and professional responsibility.

Contents

Preface

While the fundamental principles of medical ethics remain firmly grounded, with the rapid advances in technology, medical ethics has undergone necessary changes to adapt to contemporary healthcare. As medical innovations advance at unprecedented speed, healthcare systems face mounting complexity. Clinicians, patients, families, and policymakers confront ethical dilemmas that resist simple resolution.

This book addresses the ethical challenges across three critical domains. First, emerging technologies, particularly artificial intelligence and personalized medicine, raise fundamental questions about clinical judgment, patient autonomy, and equitable access to innovation. Second, decision-making under uncertainty tests traditional ethical frameworks, whether in parents navigating complex pediatric interventions or in clinicians balancing patient safety with autonomy in the use of restraints. Third, structural forces, including economic pressures, resource scarcity, and social determinants of health, shape clinical practice in ways that challenge medicine's foundational ethical commitments.

The twelve chapters in this volume provide ethical analyses grounded in real-world practice that acknowledge that ethical decision-making in healthcare rarely involves choosing between right and wrong but rather navigating competing goods, uncertain outcomes, and value conflicts that resist algorithmic resolution.

This book serves healthcare professionals, bioethicists, policymakers, and students seeking frameworks for ethical reasoning that honor both principled analysis and the complexities of clinical practice.

Thomas F. Heston, MD, MSc
Clinical Assistant Professor,
Department of Family Medicine,
University of Washington,
Seattle, United States of America

Clinical Associate Professor,
Department of Medical Education and Clinical Sciences,
Washington State University,
Spokane, WA USA

Chapter 1

Perspective Chapter: With Love as Our Guide – A Parent's Reflection on Complex Medical Decision-Making, Hindsight, and the Limits of Science

Noel Boyle

Abstract

Nearly twenty-five years ago, confronting conflicting surgical opinions, we decided our son would have epilepsy surgery. The decision was well justified, the medical care he received was excellent, and the surgery seemed to save his life. Four years later, thanks to his mother's diligence, genetic testing confirmed the diagnosis of Dravet syndrome. While securing suitable treatment, the diagnosis also meant that epilepsy surgery had been objectively harmful, not beneficial. In this chapter, I tell the story of Ciaran's epilepsy surgery, exploring the complex and seemingly contradictory viewpoints from which to consider whether he should have had surgery. I contrast the physician's imperative to provide a high standard of care with the parental focus on the child's flourishing. I consider the role of hindsight and the nature of medical regret. The result, I hope, is a philosophical narrative from the extremes of high-stakes medical decision-making, and a story of parental love at the frontiers of medicine.

Keywords: hemispherectomy, Dravet syndrome, conflicting surgical opinions, medical hindsight, parental role in medicine

1. Introduction: The question

Ciaran's face stretched tight and shiny from swelling. His skin seemed like fragile paper. He was only two years old. Immediately post-op, he had two black eyes. Six hours later, we couldn't even see his eyes. The swelling in his eyelids, cheeks, and even his forehead had cocooned his eyeballs, hiding the bruising near his eye sockets. Under his chin, chafed folds of skin started to break out in a yeast infection. His head seemed inflated, as if about to pop. Wrapped layers of gauze fit like a snug helmet. A bundling of wires came out the back of his head. Electroencephalogram (EEG) recordings were displayed on a bedside monitor. He was on video camera. That was near the beginning, when things were still going well. The hard part wouldn't start for another week.

In 2002, my two-year-old son had the left half of his brain removed. The need for epilepsy surgery, even hemispherectomy, is often medically uncontroversial. Second opinions usually reinforce recommendations from other epilepsy surgery centers. Parental decisions, though devastating, are generally clear. Surgery usually goes as planned. Rarely do later tests fundamentally alter the diagnosis. None of that is true in Ciaran's case.

Should Ciaran have had epilepsy surgery? It depends. Is it a question about the medical evidence available at the time, or a question about the whole factual situation? Is the question addressed to the physicians who performed the surgery, or to me and Jessica, his parents, who made the final decision? Ciaran cannot use language; can the question still be addressed to him? Aside from the "about what" and the "to whom" of the question, there is also the "of when." Is the question merely about the past, or is it asked with an eye toward an emerging future? Whether Ciaran should have had epilepsy surgery depends on what is meant by the question. The answer is known, but it isn't simple. A lot of life is like that, and the story of Ciaran's epilepsy surgery displays universal structures of uncertainty, regret, and hindsight. On account of parental decision-making at the extremes, it is mostly a story about love.

2. Hemispherectomy

The first way to ask whether Ciaran should have had epilepsy surgery is from within the epistemic situation in which the decision was made, considering only what was known at the time and the reasons the decision was made at the time.

Starting this story at the beginning, Jessica and I met in college and fell in love while studying philosophy together. We married in 1998, a couple of years after graduation. Ciaran was born the next year, in early November of 1999. Despite complications at birth necessitating a C-section, he thrived for six months. At Christmas time, I even told my sister-in-law that parenting was easier than I'd expected. I was twenty-six years old at the time; Jessica was twenty-eight. In May of 2000, at six months old, Ciaran suddenly started having catastrophic seizures. His first seizure lasted forty-five minutes. The second, two days later and of a different type, lasted nearly an hour. Despite coming under the care of a pediatric neurologist specializing in epilepsy, from that point until surgery, every four or five days Ciaran would have a seizure so terrible that the medication required to stop it was enough to suppress his urge to breathe, often necessitating a couple of hours of mechanical breathing. Between such instances of *status epilepticus,* he was having as many as 400 little seizures a day. Seizures were an immediate and growing threat to his life. They terrorized him daily. The apparent wreckage was growing, as his cognitive developmental progress began to slow within weeks of the first seizures, and he was noticeably regressing by his first birthday.

Medicaid covered a trip to the Mayo Clinic, where they "diagnosed" him with an "idiopathic, cryptogenic, and refractory seizure disorder." The use of such language hides normal medical ignorance in fancy terminology designed to dazzle and distract from the human limitations of medical practitioners. In direct language, the Mayo concluded only that they didn't know the underlying cause of the seizures, they didn't know what triggered particular seizures, and they didn't know how to stop any of it.

In spite of the seizures, Ciaran's tenacious and mischievous personality emerged. When he was not being terrorized by seizures, he loved to snuggle (he still does). He enjoyed good food. Most of all, he loved to run and climb. Recklessly rambunctious on the neighborhood playground equipment, he had a categorical faith that I would catch him when he jumped. He even recovered from traumatic seizures more quickly than we did. ER doctors entering Ciaran's room an hour after a life-threatening seizure often found a kid climbing all over the room, barely contained by two exhausted and clearly traumatized parents. Sometimes, they thought they must be in the wrong room. One memorable morning, Ciaran was admitted to the pediatric ICU on a ventilator, only to be discharged later the same day after gleefully bouncing in his wheelchair, throwing macaroni and cheese at the glass doors. In 2001, when his younger brother was born, Ciaran was Teagin's first hospital visitor. The visit was unplanned; Ciaran was supposed to stay home with Grandma. Instead, Ciaran made his usual dramatic entrance through the ER. By the time I got from the maternity unit to the ER, the seizure was already over. Soon afterward, despite protestations from the maternity unit staff, Jess came down to check on him, leaving Teagin in his aunt's arms. Ciaran was soon discharged, and we brought him to meet Teagin and spend a few hours with us in the maternity unit, snuggled up as a family of four.

Of course, we tried everything else before considering surgery. For idiopathic seizure disorders, surgery is the treatment of last resort for good reasons. The brutality of epilepsy surgery is inescapable. The goal is to find the part of the brain causing the seizures and, with scalpel and suction, take it out. The operation is planned in two stages. The first involves sawing through the skull to remove one side, cutting through the dura enveloping the brain, and placing dozens of electrodes directly on areas of the brain suspected to be generating seizures. Those electrodes are attached to wires that come out of a hole in the back of the head. Data from the electrodes are used in the second surgical stage a couple of days later, determining the precise areas of the brain to be excised, labeled, and sent to the laboratory in jars.

Jessica and I decided he would have this surgery. We cannot pass responsibility for the decision onto the physicians because they could not agree among themselves. A nearly identical month-long surgical evaluation at one of the nation's best pediatric epilepsy centers concluded with a strong recommendation for surgery as soon as possible, it being his only hope. A nearly identical month-long surgical evaluation at one of the nation's other best pediatric epilepsy centers concluded that he would not benefit from surgery and that there was no real hope. There was nothing wrong with either medical opinion; the disagreement was reasonable, a matter of different analyses of an agreed-upon set of well-documented facts. The epileptologists leading the two evaluations even spoke privately about Ciaran's case. The reason the doctors could not agree among themselves was not that Ciaran needed better or more diligent doctors. There weren't better doctors.

The process could be considered an exemplar of Lainie Friedman Ross's influential model of shared parent–physician decision-making, known as "constrained parental autonomy" [1, 2]. Physicians presented us with a small set of medically reasonable options, and we had the autonomy necessary to make the value-informed choice that was best for our family. Ross criticizes common views that define the "best interest of the patient" in ways that are reducible to medical science and isolated from cultural and personal values [1, 2]. Ciaran's case exemplifies Ross's critiques. Medical judgments are not themselves value-neutral, and when they try to be, they can entirely lose their capacity to inform decision-making. The bioethical literature is replete with examples of parent's failures to meet their obligations under shared decision-making. Ciaran highlights what I suspect is a more common problem: The inability of medical science to fill the role it ascribes to itself under such models.

After all, our situation seemed absurd. There were no discernible medical grounds on which to choose between the incompatible recommendations of the medical teams, and yet a medical decision was urgently needed. We were left to adjudicate the medical dispute because we are his parents, a title requiring no training whatsoever. Precisely because the experts couldn't agree, it seemed that nonexperts had to decide instead. This was not shared decision-making except by virtue of deeply personal and downright philosophical conversations we were blessed to occasionally have with Ciaran's local pediatric neurologist. The medical establishment, inevitably divided within itself due to the inherent limitations of science, vacated its role in decision-making. This was a parental, not shared, decision.

Of course, as Ciaran's parents, it is our legal and moral right to choose which qualified medical team will oversee his care. That is a sacred right and an important one to assert. It is not always respected. Despite appearances, it is not absurd that it was our decision to make; it was perfectly ordinary. What made the situation absurd were the unfathomable stakes in the exercise of our ordinary right. In choosing which medical center we would schedule Ciaran's continuing care with, we were also deciding whether his brain would remain whole. Parents make consequential decisions on behalf of their young children all the time; our decision was no different in kind, but only by a large degree. The rights of parents are unusual and are best understood as obligations to attempt to secure their children's genuine flourishing.

From Ciaran's first seizures, we took our obligation as seriously as we could. John Freeman's *Seizures and Epilepsy in Childhood: A Guide for Parents*, written with his Johns Hopkins colleagues, Eileen Vining and Diana Pillas, was everything for us that such a book might hope to be. Advising parents on thinking through the surgical decision, they offer what we call the Mirror Test: "If surgery is unsuccessful, if the child continues to have seizures, if there are complications of surgery and the child is more impaired, or dead, you still have to brush your teeth, look yourself in the eye, and be able to state with great conviction that you made the best decision possible for you and your child" [3]. Epilepsy surgery is irreversible. There are always things that are simply unknowable at the time of surgery, and future events can have unpredictable consequences. No one was asking us to be gods. Yet, it was our imperative to proceed in the right way. Our love for Ciaran, and our love for each other, was our guide. Holistic and critical evaluation of the knowable facts was our task. Only a mutual decision, collaboratively reached in full reciprocal relationship, would do. As philosophy majors, we had the best possible preparation for making such impossible decisions.

We read all the medical reports. We studied as much of the relevant science as we could. We learned the basics of how to interpret EEGs. We tried to read the relevant medical journal articles that were coauthored by Ciaran's doctors. We grasped subtle differences in the relative value different epileptologists give to different kinds of medical evidence. We came to understand *why* there were no purely medical or scientific grounds to resolve the physicians' disagreements. We endlessly discussed the differences between the physicians' clinical styles and their different approaches to risk assessment. Initially, we disagreed with one another. Knowing we would either pass the Mirror Test together or we were each likely to fail it alone, we treated our disagreement as a blessing. Neither would be convinced until both were.

It took time. Working through our own disagreement lovingly and intellectually, we kept asking ourselves what Ciaran would think if he could understand everything involved in our decision. Our question was not "What would I want if it were me?" or "What would Jess want if it were her?" Those two might be different from one another, and neither seemed particularly relevant. We sought what care ethicist Nel Noddings called "motivational displacement," shifting our motivations to Ciaran's interests [4]. We wanted to know whether Ciaran would choose to have the surgery if he were able to make a fully informed choice. To the extent possible, we wanted Ciaran's perspective to be central, and his values to be determinative. Contrary to the common Kantian assumption made by Ross and others, it is dangerously misguided dogma to suggest that the child's point of view is only a relevant consideration to the extent that the child is autonomous or even capable of developing autonomy. We should, instead, adopt what philosopher Eva Feder Kittay calls the "sufficiency condition" and recognize that merely being human confers full moral worth on a person and, thereby, establishes the centrality of *their own* considerations to *their* medical care [5, 6].

Puzzling over the methodological challenges associated with trying to speak for Ciaran as an individual person, our reflections repeatedly circled back to his exuberant thirst for life, his determined nature, and his ebullient joy. Slowly, we came to recognize that Ciaran's personality aligned better with the kind of risk assessment done by the team recommending surgery. It would involve terrible suffering and trauma, for him and for us, but it might give him a chance. He wanted a chance to have a life.

Should Ciaran have had epilepsy surgery? Some might insist on an answer at this point, from inside the epistemic situation in which the decision was made. The rest of this chapter describes things that weren't knowable when the surgery started. In one sense, it isn't fair to evaluate a decision based on what couldn't be known when it was made. In a more compelling sense, however, fairness demands that we consider how things turned out for Ciaran.

Epilepsy surgery did not go as hoped. The first operation went as planned, though giving robustly informed consent to surgery is very different from actually encountering your child's severe medical injuries. The mental images, described in this chapter's opening, are forever seared in my imagination. Surgeons used data gathered in the days after the first surgery to determine the precise parts of his temporal and frontal lobes to remove in the second surgery, which initially seemed successful as well. After several days of sound healing, seizures suddenly started again and did not stop. Ciaran developed *continual partial epilepsy*, an ever-continuing and ongoing seizure. Starting with a little twitch in his right foot, convulsions grew slowly but steadily, marching up his body and coming to encompass his right leg and then his right arm as well. Seconds after his face started twitching, both sides of his whole body suddenly began convulsing in a violent episode of *status epilepticus*. Intervention with large doses of Ativan settled everything but a little twitch in his right foot. In unrelenting eight- to ten-hour cycles, the pattern repeated. On a whiteboard in Ciaran's room, we tracked the cycle for nine days.

We had been clearly told that the need for more extensive surgical resection was a possible complication. Epilepsy surgery often involves a balance between excising as much of the brain as is necessary while leaving as much as possible intact. We understood that Ciaran's case was unusually complicated and that his risks were, therefore, unusually high. Before considering more surgery, of course, extensive new diagnostic testing was needed. Throughout the process, we lived at the Ronald McDonald House, where eight-month-old Teagin became such a familiarly joyous presence that the Director declared him the house's Official Smiling Baby. Inside the hospital, we held Ciaran while he screamed as if being tortured when they placed scalp electrodes directly on the twice-cut-through surgical scar running across the top of his head. The data indicated erratic seizure activity throughout the remaining parts of the left hemisphere. The lead epileptologist said he had never encountered a brain so prone to seizing in his twenty-five-year career. After urgent but careful deliberation, they determined he needed to have the rest of the left side of his brain removed. He howled in abject terror as we carried him into the surgical prep unit for the third time. I still feel sick when I think about it. We learned later that Teagin wouldn't eat that day either.

After hemispherectomy, Ciaran never went into *status epilepticus* again, though a moderate and manageable seizure disorder persisted. He responded enthusiastically to physical therapy and was soon walking again. Our highest hope was that he would develop a capacity to use language, though he never did. In time, he had difficult setbacks. A year after the hemispherectomy, he needed a shunt to manage hydrocephalus caused by the surgery. Soon, he became entirely reliant on a feeding tube as well. But he lived. In time, we found better treatment for his seizure disorder, and he thrived through puberty. In his late teenage years, orthopedic problems permanently took from him the ability to walk, though he can still scoot around on his own. Terrible pneumonias in early adulthood resulted in a tracheostomy, and today he needs a ventilator at night. In 2022, he was able to earn a special education diploma from Nashville public schools, where he joyously attended the Harris-Hillman School for twelve years. Today, he is twenty-five and is still able to live with us at home. During the week, he is under the loving care of skilled home care nurses, particularly Gordon. On the weekends, we care for him ourselves. All in all, he is mostly happy and able to flourish in his own way. He is living a life.

Should Ciaran have had epilepsy surgery? Yes. The surgery was both medically justified and successful by its own stated goals, though imperfectly so. Our fundamental purpose was achieved, but not our highest goals. Enormous costs were justified by existential benefits. Is that all there is to it? The answer is still only measured in light of what we knew then. What we know now changes everything.

3. Dravet syndrome

In 2006, four years after epilepsy surgery, Jessica learned about Dravet syndrome while searching the Internet in the slim hope that she might find the underlying cause of Ciaran's seizures. Parroting things I'd heard from physicians, I told her that there likely was no answer to be found. Even if she did succeed, it would almost certainly change neither Ciaran's treatment nor his prognosis. Jessica understood that, but she wanted to put a name to what did this to our child. When she encountered Dravet syndrome, the description largely matched the early course of

Ciaran's illness. Jessica suggested a diagnosis of Dravet syndrome to Ciaran's neurologists, who were skeptical but intrigued. Pressing the point, Jessica was able to get a case summary to Dr. Dravet herself. Upon learning that a child who had undergone hemispherectomy might have Dravet syndrome, Dr. Dravet was fascinated, as she believed the situation would be unique. Eventually, she made the formal diagnosis herself during a clinic visit where she evaluated Ciaran on the sidelines of a conference in Minnesota. Subsequent genetic testing confirmed beyond doubt that the underlying cause of Ciaran's seizures is a *de* novo mutation to his SCN1A gene. Ciaran's mom outperformed the medical establishment.

The 2007 confirmation of the Dravet syndrome diagnosis *entirely* changed Ciaran's treatment and prognosis. At the time, his seizures were worsening again. When insurance cut off speech therapy services for lack of demonstrable progress, we wept long and bitterly with his speech therapist, Eileen. That her heroic efforts left her feeling defeated was symbolic of that period of time as a whole. Ciaran's hospitalizations grew longer and more frequent. He was increasingly lethargic, dwindling. He hadn't smiled in years. After discussions with the intensive care staff in 2006, we signed a DNR order and prearranged a funeral for our seven-year-old, explaining it all to his five-year-old brother as best we could.

The diagnosis of Dravet determined that most of the anti-seizure medications he was given as an infant made his seizures worse. They were sodium channel blockers and thereby accelerated seizures in patients with Dravet syndrome. As doctors thought they were responding to the rapid progression of his seizure disorder, their treatments were actually the cause of the rapid progression. The upside to that disturbing realization was enormous: suitable treatment. Within a couple of years, always following empirical medical science, we started giving him CBD derived from cannabis (illegally at first, but now covered by his medical insurance). His seizures abated, and his energy soared. He settled into life as a student at the Harris-Hillman School. He smiled again. He smiled a lot.

With the diagnosis of Dravet syndrome, we also learned that the underlying cause of his epilepsy was not located in one specific part of his brain more than in another. Had the diagnosis been made during the surgical evaluation, it would have ended all possible consideration of surgery. Epilepsy surgery was inconceivably traumatic and unspeakably painful. The hemispherectomy caused a permanent visual impairment and cost Ciaran control over the right side of his body. No one can explain to him what happened or why. A few days after the hemispherectomy, he had to be restrained because he was using his healthy left arm to savagely slam his unresponsive right arm against the crib rails. Had he been diagnosed with Dravet syndrome in time, none of it would have happened.

Should Ciaran have had epilepsy surgery? Both medical teams missed the diagnosis, and neither would stand by their evaluations and recommendations in the face of it. Medicine got it wrong. Is that what matters in answering the question? Not if one understands the nature of medicine.

When we first met Ciaran's current neurologist in 2022, I told her that if we had never taken Ciaran to a neurologist and had just given him weed instead, hoping for the best, he would be able to walk on his own, eat and drink, use the bathroom, and could very well have command of a couple dozen words. I elaborated on how little neurology understands the disease mechanisms it treats compared to every other branch of medicine, except for its notorious cousin, psychiatry. I told her that my nickname for neurologists is "head scratchers." (They scratch Ciaran's head and then, in response, they look at each other and scratch their own.) I promised Ciaran, and myself, that I wouldn't hold back. Ciaran needs his neurologist to understand what the limits of medical knowledge have cost him. I need that. She was gracious and agreed that medical humility is particularly important for neurologists. She even conceded that I was right about the cannabis. If we had taken Ciaran to the weed guy instead of a neurologist, he would be better off today, "*given what the diagnosis turned out to be*."

It was an honest, warm, and nuanced defense of her profession. Doctors work from the medical facts in front of them. Whether some treatment constitutes good care, whether it was good medicine, *is* a question locked in the epistemic situation of the moment. When we evaluate medical decisions only with the benefit of hindsight, we are expecting physicians to be gods, and we will eventually consider them all to have been monsters instead. Ciaran's doctors, *all of them*, did an exceptional job practicing medicine. They are dedicated professionals, infused with compassion and courage. I am deeply grateful for what they did to save our son. Extraordinary human beings, my admiration for them is almost boundless.

Jessica and I are not physicians, and the parental role is different. Of course, parents also cannot reasonably be asked to do more than make the best decision they can, based on what it is possible for them to know at the time. If we had given cannabis to Ciaran as an infant instead of following the advice of qualified neurologists, he would rightly have been removed from our care so that he could get "genuine medicine" instead (regardless of the fact that everyone had the "Harmful Poison" and "Helpful Medicine" categories backward at the time). We did what parents are supposed to do, giving robustly informed consent to treatments recommended by certified professional physicians. In fact, we were privileged to be able to do an unusually good job as his parents.

Our parental decision still passes Freeman's Mirror Test. Even in hindsight, we state "with great conviction" that we made "the best decision possible." Moreover, we still state it together. I would not know how to live with myself if I believed that what happened to Ciaran was the result of our failure as his parents. I don't have to. We did the best we could have done. But the Mirror Test doesn't capture the difference between medical and parental decision-making.

A physician should be satisfied if they've practiced excellent medicine, whatever the outcome. Speaking as a parent, whether I do an excellent job as a parent is secondary. How things go for my children is what matters to me. I refuse to seek comfort in the fact that we made the best decision we could. Seeking such comfort feels like putting my own sense of parental adequacy above Ciaran's objective well-being. I am not saying we are blameworthy or at fault. We are not. We had bad moral luck, as Nagel called it [8], but we were not blameworthy. If we abandoned Ciaran, we would be at fault. If we refused to decide among legitimate medical opinions and turned to faith healing instead, we would be blameworthy. At the actual moment of our choice, there was no moral fault (or praise) in either decision we might have made. Nevertheless, another course of action would have been better for Ciaran.

Should Ciaran have had epilepsy surgery? No. People with Dravet syndrome should never have epilepsy surgery. Objectively, the surgery harmed Ciaran, rather than benefiting him. That which ended up in a jar should have stayed in his head. Inescapably, that is the primary answer to the question. I will never reconcile myself to that fact, and I do not want to. Instead, I've found a kind of peace living in the irreconcilability. That which cannot be allowed to happen also cannot be made to have not happened.

In 1978, French neurologist Charlotte Dravet noticed similarities in a group of infant patients she was caring for. It was probably only because of earlier advances in the treatment of pediatric epilepsy that these children were able to live and thrive enough for Dravet to observe their salient similarities. She proposed that the pattern noted in this group of patients was a distinct epilepsy, calling it severe myoclonic epilepsy of infancy (SMEI). The clinical pattern Dravet described was soon identified with specific genetic mutations. Her discovery of a new seizure disorder was gradually recognized, and it was eventually renamed in her honor [7, 8]. Today, in 2025, students learn about Dravet syndrome in medical school, frequently mispronouncing it by vocalizing the silent 't' at the end of her name. When an infant with Dravet syndrome arrives at a research hospital today, the fellow in pediatric neurology will probably be able to make the diagnosis at the first clinic visit. There is fault if the diagnosis is missed after a thorough evaluation overseen by the attending: from an observation by an extraordinary healer in a Parisian clinic to inclusion in the standard medical school curriculum, in only two generations.

Ciaran was born almost exactly halfway between those two points in time. Borrowing Hannah Arendt's phrase from a different context [9], Ciaran's surgical evaluation took place between the past and the future of Dravet syndrome, manifesting both a "no longer" that was still passing and a "not yet" that was yet to arrive. It is the presence of both of these in Ciaran's experience of Dravet syndrome that is ultimately irreconcilable. How can the past and future of a disease exist inside one person?

In the year prior to his 2002 hemispherectomy, Ciaran had been evaluated at Children's Hospital of Michigan's epilepsy monitoring unit for over a month, spread across multiple occasions, supplemented by numerous clinic visits. He spent two weeks being evaluated at Cleveland Clinic's epilepsy monitoring unit, and he stayed nearly a full month at the Mayo Clinic's. We sent his records to be evaluated by the pediatric epilepsy surgery team at Johns Hopkins, the best in the world. (I called Hopkins to confirm they'd received the files and was star struck when Dr. Freeman himself answered the phone.) Through all of that, Ciaran practically lived at DeVos Children's Hospital, where he and his brother were born, where they saved his life innumerable times in the emergency department, and we were on a first-name basis with most of the staff. Through all of that, no one mentioned Dravet syndrome. I don't think any of them had heard of it yet, even though it had already been two decades since Dravet's first landmark paper and sixteen years since the publication of her work in English.

I confess bitterness that Ciaran was evaluated at centers with reputations built on providing care on the frontlines of medical research, and he had the surgery anyway. The correct diagnosis was, quite literally, already on the shelf in their library. How dare they miss it! I call my bitterness a confession because it is not reasonable; it does not stand up to scrutiny. The diagnosis was completely missed by too many physicians, each too distinguished in the field for me to reasonably conclude that there was fault or medical failure in any of them missing the diagnosis. If Ciaran needed better doctors, or doctors who did a better job, anger might be justified. What he needed was for medicine to progress faster than it did, and feeling bitter that it did not is neither rational nor healthy. Instead, I try to set aside bitterness and dwell in the strange comfort of permanent irreconcilability. Like medicine, however, I am a work in progress.

4. Conclusion: The answer

The premise of the question seems to be that Ciaran's life story could have been different, and that an alternate version would not have included epilepsy surgery. It implies that things might have been different, without postulating a specific alternative. Jessica and I could not have arrived at a different final decision without some kind of difference in the background facts available to us. But if the question offers license to imagine changes in our background knowledge, I'll soon be noting that we should have booked flights to Paris after his second seizure. Moreover, imagining all that might have been, no parent would say their child's life should include epilepsy, let alone epilepsy surgery. What should have been different is that Ciaran's SCN1A gene should not have mutated. If I could change anything, it would be that.

Thus, the question is not quite what it seems to be; the answer that matters is not about how the past might have been different. The past can't be undone. The answer that matters, the form of the question that ultimately matters, is about what is true today.

Ciaran survived long enough to be diagnosed with Dravet syndrome only because gifted healers dedicate their careers to being respiratory therapists, paramedics, emergency department nurses, epileptologists, nurses, neurosurgeons, and so on. Ciaran was diagnosed with Dravet syndrome only because his mother kept looking for a diagnostic answer when no one else knew how. Absent either of those, we could not ask the question and know to be troubled by its answers. While Ciaran's epilepsy surgery cannot be changed, what has changed is that no family confronting Dravet syndrome will ever again be asked such a question.

Acknowledgments

Thanks to Ginger Osborn and Charmion Gustke, both colleagues at Belmont University, for their invaluable comments on an earlier draft. Thanks also to Eva Feder Kittay for her encouragement and suggestions.

Author details

Noel Boyle
Department of Philosophy, Belmont University, Nashville, TN, United States

*Address all correspondence to: noel.boyle@belmont.edu

References

[1] Ross LF. Children, Families, and Health Care Decision Making. Oxford (UK): Clarendon Press; 1998.

[2] Ross LF. The philosophical underpinning of the family for pediatric decision-making. Pediatric Clinics of North America. 2024;**71**(1):27–37.

[3] Freeman JM, Vining E, and Pillas D. Seizures and Epilepsy in Childhood: A Guide for Parents, 2nd ed. Baltimore, Maryland: Johns Hopkins University Press; 1997. pp. 186.

[4] Noddings N. Caring: A Feminine Approach to Ethics and Moral Education. Berkeley: University of California Press; 1984.

[5] Kittay EF. Getting from here to there: Claiming justice for the severely disabled. In Rhodes R, Battin MP, Silvers A, editors. Medicine and Social Justice: Essays on the Distribution of Health Care. 2nd ed. New York: Oxford University Press; 2012. pp. 314–324.

[6] Kittay EF. Why human difference is critical to a conception of moral standing: An argument for the sufficiency of being human for full moral status. The Journal of Philosophy of Disability. 2021;**1**:79–103.

[7] Dravet C, and Guerrini R. Dravet Syndrome. Esher, Surrey, UK: John Libbey Eurotext; 2011.

[8] Nagel T. Moral Luck. In Mortal Questions Thomas Nagel. Cambridge (UK): Cambridge University Press; 1979. p. 24–38.

[9] Arendt H. Between past and Future: Eight Exercises in Political Thought. Revised ed. New York: Penguin; 2006.

Chapter 2

The Ethical Prerogative to Eradicate Measles and Rubella

David N. Durrheim

Abstract

No vaccine has been more effective in reducing infectious disease mortality, especially among children, than the measles-containing vaccine. The measles vaccine is one of the most cost-effective public health measures. Exhaustive reviews of biological, technical, economic, and programmatic evidence have concluded that measles can and should be eradicated. By including the rubella antigen in the measles-containing vaccine, disabling congenital rubella syndrome would contemporaneously also be eradicated. There are compelling ethical arguments for committing to and completing measles and rubella eradication. The principle of beneficence mandates that national governments and the international community have a duty of care to ensure that current and future cohorts of children all enjoy this ultimate protection against measles and rubella viruses. The rule of rescue places an obligation on global decision-makers to set an eradication goal and invest adequately to 'rescue' current and future generations of children facing avoidable death, as the attendant 'sacrifice' is not excessive. The collateral benefits of strengthening primary health care delivery to all communities and enhancing disease surveillance everywhere, using measles as a tracer, are potentially enormous. As deaths particularly affect young children, the fair innings argument is another strong motivation for completing the eradication journey. Reciprocity places a burden on wealthier nations to support developing countries towards achieving this shared goal. Measles, rubella, and congenital rubella syndrome eradication should be completed to ensure that future generations of children do not live under the shadow of preventable childhood death and lifelong disability.

Keywords: measles, rubella, congenital rubella syndrome, eradication, elimination, immunisation, vaccination, vaccine, ethics, beneficence, rule of rescue, sanctity of life, justice, equity

1. Introduction

'There can be no keener revelation of a society's soul than the way in which it treats its children.' Nelson Mandela

Throughout history, the measles virus has exacted an enormous death toll, particularly on young children and across all age-groups when first introduced into virgin populations [1, 2]. For example, in 1980 alone, six years after the Expanded Programme on Immunization was launched to increase global uptake of vaccines in children, an estimated 2.6 million children died due to measles and its complications [3]. In wealthy countries, complications, particularly bronchopneumonia, diarrhoea, and otitis media, are common, while acute encephalitis (1 in 2,000 cases), subacute sclerosing panencephalitis (1 in 25,000 cases), and death also occur [4]. In developing countries, measles severity is even more devastating [5]. The interplay of measles infection with poor nutrition and co-infections results in a median community case fatality ratio approaching 4%, and reported death rates have exceeded 40% in some very high-risk settings, such as refugee camps with low vaccination coverage [6]. Many additional deaths result from the array of viral and bacterial infections that exploit measles virus infection–induced immune amnesia, which persists for many months following measles infection [7].

The rapid increase in global measles vaccine coverage had a profound impact on measles-related mortality, with the goal of a 50% reduction in measles deaths by 2005, compared with 1999, being achieved [8]. A fifty-year review of the Expanded Program on Immunization found that measles vaccination was the single greatest contributor to lives saved by vaccination; 93.7 million deaths had been averted by measles vaccination, with a staggering 5.7 billion years of life saved [8]. Measles vaccination accounted for 60.8% of the 154.0 million total lives saved by vaccination over the five decades.

2. Disease eradication criteria

The eradication of an infectious disease – the permanent reduction to zero of the worldwide incidence of infection caused by a specific agent as a result of deliberate efforts – is considered the pinnacle of public health achievement [9]. This possibility was first envisaged by Edward Jenner, who commented after the initial success of his smallpox vaccination: 'This practice would wipe out this scourge from the face of the earth' [10]. Jenner was correct, with smallpox eradication declared at the 33rd World Health Assembly in 1980 [11].

Despite numerous other disease eradication attempts – hookworm, malaria, yellow fever, yaws, polio – no other human infectious disease has yet been eradicated, despite the footprint of each of these diseases being dramatically reduced through eradication and control efforts. These attempts have proven invaluable in identifying the characteristics of human infectious diseases that make them amenable – or not – to eradication. Critical success elements include: (i) an effective intervention – most often a vaccine – must be available to interrupt transmission of the infectious agent; (ii) practical diagnostic tools with sufficient sensitivity and specificity to reliably detect infection should exist; and (iii) humans should be essential for the lifecycle of the agent, which should not have any other vertebrate reservoir or be able to amplify in the environment [12]. Demonstrated success of the eradication strategy in a large geographic area or region is predictive of the likelihood of eradication success [13].

The International Task Force for Disease Eradication recommended a careful review of three broad considerations before embarking on eradication: (i) biological and technical feasibility (as listed above); (ii) costs and benefits; and (iii) societal and political considerations [14]. As thinking has evolved, two further characteristics deserve explicit consideration. Firstly, the infection should induce life-long immunity [15]. Secondly, reflecting on the success of smallpox eradication, high-quality surveillance is essential for focusing end-game efforts [16].

3. Measles and rubella eradication feasibility

In 2010, an expert advisory committee, chaired by the author, was convened by the World Health Organization (WHO) in Washington, DC, to assess the feasibility of measles eradication. The panel concluded that eradication was indeed biologically, technically, and operationally feasible with existing tools, as demonstrated in the Region of the Americas, with endemic measles transmission declared eliminated in 2002, and in countries in every other region [17]. The expert advisory committee concluded that measles can and should be eradicated; eradication by 2020 was feasible if measurable progress was made towards existing 2015 measles mortality reduction targets; measles eradication activities should occur in the context of strengthening routine immunisation services; and measles eradication activities should be used to accelerate control and elimination of rubella and congenital rubella syndrome.

Later that year, WHO's Strategic Advisory Group of Experts on Immunization declared that 'measles can and should be eradicated' [18]. All six WHO Regions established goals to eliminate measles on or before 2020, so there was a de facto eradication goal if all Regions delivered on their commitment. The World Health Assembly adopted the goal of achieving measles and rubella elimination in at least five WHO Regions by 2020 when it endorsed the Global Vaccine Action Plan in May 2012 [19]. This visionary initiative aimed to extend the benefits of vaccination to all people, everywhere.

Rubella elimination is considered highly feasible, as almost all countries use combined measles-rubella-containing vaccines, and the rubella virus is much less infectious than the measles virus, requiring about 85% coverage with a single rubella vaccine dose in each birth cohort to achieve elimination, compared to the 95% coverage with two measles vaccine doses required for measles elimination [20, 21].

4. Current global measles and rubella situation

Unfortunately, despite having WHO regional goals, the lack of a galvanising global eradication goal with attendant appropriate resource investment has resulted in erratic progress towards measles and rubella elimination.

The increase in global first-dose measles immunisation coverage from 72% to 86% during 2000–2019, and a concurrent increase in global second-dose measles immunisation coverage from 18% in 2000 to 71% in 2019, averted an estimated 25.5 million measles deaths [22]. By 2022, the estimated number of deaths prevented by measles vaccination had risen to approximately 57 million worldwide [23].

With strong regional leadership, over half of all member states have been verified to have achieved rubella elimination, and endemic rubella transmission has not been re-established in any verified country to date [24]. In 2023, 84 countries and territories were verified to have sustained elimination of measles, which is a phenomenal achievement [25]. However, without a global target, this success will be difficult to sustain, as evidenced by 13 countries in the Americas, Western Pacific, and European regions that experienced reestablished measles virus circulation after previously being verified to have achieved endemic measles elimination.

Following a decade during which global first-dose measles immunisation coverage stagnated at 85% – leaving nearly 20 million children in every annual birth cohort unprotected against measles – and inadequate second-dose coverage to guarantee enduring immunity, the COVID-19 pandemic further hindered progress towards measles and rubella elimination. Existing perilous measles immunity gaps were widened due to delayed vaccination campaigns and suspended routine immunisation activities [26]. The resulting global resurgence perpetuates the five-yearly cycle of massive worldwide measles waves with surges in preventable deaths (2014, 2019/20, 2024/25). This wretched epidemiological situation is inevitable without a true commitment to measles eradication [27].

Over 30,000 babies are born every year with disabling congenital rubella syndrome [28]. To accelerate progress towards measles and rubella eradication, rubella vaccine introduction should be implemented in the remaining countries where it is not currently part of the routine immunisation schedule without delay [29]. Using wide-age-range immunisation campaigns with combined measles-rubella vaccines for rubella vaccine introduction will not only eliminate congenital rubella syndrome but also provide a broad buffer of measles immunity in the age group that contributes greatly to its spread.

5. The economics of eradication

The added effort required to reach every community and child with measles and rubella-containing vaccines necessary for achieving eradication will have associated substantial costs. The funding and human resources required, particularly in resource-poor settings, will, of necessity, result in opportunity costs to local health services, and wealthy donors will also be required to contribute. However, if eradication is achieved, then impressive savings will accrue directly through vaccination doses that are no longer necessary and treatment costs averted.

The costs of responding to and containing measles outbreaks are enormous. Even small outbreaks can be enormously disruptive and place a huge burden on public health services, whether in wealthy or developing countries [30–33].

The measles-containing vaccine is one of the most cost-effective public health interventions. The return on investment is $58 in direct illness treatment costs saved for every $1 invested in immunisation [34]. It has been estimated that the eradication of measles and rubella could save at least US$10 billion per year in treatment costs, even without considering the benefits of preventing lost productivity and potential savings from reduced vaccination [35]. A recent update of this analysis, from a US perspective alone, estimated even greater net benefits from achieving measles and rubella eradication [36].

This should not be surprising. A $300 million effort succeeded in completely eradicating smallpox in less than a decade, and the United States, the largest contributor to that program, has recouped that level of investment every 26 days since eradication, in funds not spent on vaccinations and the costs of treating new smallpox cases [37].

6. The rights of the child and equity

When the Convention on the Rights of the Child was adopted by the United Nations (UN) General Assembly in 1989, it was the only international legally binding instrument to include all human rights, including political, economic, sociocultural, and civil rights [38]. Global acceptance has been remarkable, with all UN member states, except Somalia and the United States, having ratified the Convention.

Article 6 (Survival and Development) states: *Children have the right to live. Governments should ensure that children survive and develop healthily.* As detailed above, immunisation against childhood diseases is considered one of the most effective public health measures for realising this worthy goal, and measles immunisation is arguably one of the most cost-effective child survival interventions.

This requirement holds regardless of a country's development status. Article 4 (Protection of Rights) states: *Governments have a responsibility to take all available measures to ensure children's rights, in this case, access to life-saving vaccines, are respected, protected, and fulfilled*. Thus, every government has an obligation to provide all its children access to measles-rubella-containing immunisation.

Tools for ensuring equitable vaccine access exist. The Reaching Every District (RED) approach, which includes the development of local plans, linking with communities, utilising community volunteers, expanding outreach services, conducting supervisory visits, and using simple monitoring strategies, has proven effective even in challenging environments [39]. Marginalised groups, including the rural poor, migrants, and nomadic communities, are more likely to miss out on the benefits of vaccination. As these children are often at the greatest risk of severe disease due to their underlying nutritional status and have limited access to health care, reaching them with immunisation directly addresses health inequalities.

Article 24 (Health and Health Services) places an explicit equity requirement on wealthier countries: *Children have the right to good-quality health care .... Rich countries should help poorer countries achieve this*. There is a strong correlation between immunisation coverage and a country's income level [40]. Wealthy countries can make a huge difference globally by investing in this proven equity strategy.

7. Duty of care and rule to rescue

The principle of beneficence contends that every national government and the broader international community has a duty of care to ensure that current and future birth cohorts of children all enjoy the protection offered by measles- and rubella-containing vaccines to mitigate their risk of severe disease, disability, and death [41]. The strength of the duty of care prerogative depends on the availability of effective and affordable measures, which are satisfied by measles- and rubella-containing vaccines, as argued above.

The rule of rescue places an obligation on those who are able, in this case, governments and health personnel, to rescue identifiable individuals facing avoidable death if personal sacrifice is not excessive [42]. Although this principle is more generally invoked to support individual rescue efforts, it is equally valid in a global health context [43].

Beneficence is influenced by the consequences of doing nothing, the feasibility of preventing serious consequences, and the scale of sacrifice. The measles virus is unforgiving in discovering immunity gaps due to its phenomenal infectiousness, and coverage declines inevitably result in large-scale outbreaks [44]. Economic modelling has demonstrated that a coordinated campaign achieving global interruption of measles virus circulation would generate a massive return on investment, freeing up substantial finances currently required to treat hospitalised cases and respond to outbreaks [45]. However, any decrease in the level of investment will trigger a rebound of cases and deaths, with a catastrophic loss of gains. As the burden of severe disease and deaths particularly falls on young children, intergenerational equity, sometimes referred to as the 'fair innings' argument, is highly relevant [46]. The beneficence case for measles and rubella eradication is thus compelling [47].

8. Reverence for life

Albert Schweitzer, the architect of the reverence-for-life principle, contended that every life is precious: 'Ethics are responsibility without limit towards all that lives' [48]. Failing to complete the task of eradicating measles and rubella would be an unacceptable act of omission. Every child death due to measles after 2020, the date that every WHO region committed to eliminating measles, is an indictment of our shared humanity.

9. Solidarity and reciprocity

Global solidarity demands that all countries exercise good neighbourliness and optimise their own immunisation coverage to limit the risk of exporting the virus to their neighbours. As coordinated control and surveillance efforts, particularly synchronising mass vaccination campaigns, have a strong evidence base for effectiveness, this approach is strongly supported [49, 50].

Reciprocity – the 'golden rule' – entreats wealthy countries to partner with poorer countries to support them in their quest to achieve measles and rubella eradication [51].

10. Collateral benefits

Being the most contagious vaccine-preventable disease, with a highly recognisable rash, makes measles an effective tracer of populations with immunity gaps [52]. The surveillance sensitivity required for rapidly detecting, confirming, and responding to measles outbreaks allows accurate identification of specific communities missing out on measles immunisation as well as other primary health care services [53]. The strengthening of all health system building blocks; health workforce, service delivery, information, vaccine supply, cold chain, financing, and governance, at the local level, required to reach 95% of children in every community with a potent measles vaccine, is an effective means of strengthening the delivery of all other primary child health services [54–56].

11. Ethical counterviews

An ethical concern has been raised that, where eradication is claimed to have been achieved, surveillance efforts will rapidly decline, and because control measures have been relaxed or ceased, 'eradication means replacing prophylaxis and vigilance with indifference and trust' [57]. Imperfect surveillance and clandestine pathogen circulation or bio-terror release could result in devastating disease in unprotected individuals.

As very high immunisation coverage with the effective measles-containing vaccine is necessary to achieve eradication, if large numbers of individuals choose not to have themselves or their children vaccinated, inadequate coverage will thwart eradication efforts. Thus, there is unresolved tension between the public good and individual rights [58].

A theoretical concern relates to the evolutionary vacuum that would result from eradicating measles and rubella viruses. However, there is little compelling evidence to support this contention. No association between the successful smallpox eradication effort and the emergence of mpox as a human infectious disease has been proven. In countries where measles and rubella endemic circulation has been interrupted for multiple decades, there is no evidence of another virus filling the gap; in fact, while there were 18 co-circulating measles genotypes in 2003, these have steadily decreased, with only 2 genotypes detected globally since 2021, and no replacement genotypes or competing viruses have emerged [59].

12. Conclusions

All governments, health care providers, and parents have an obligation to take all reasonable measures to protect today's children and, where possible, future generations against infections that claim their lives or potentially disable them. This is particularly pertinent where a means is available which, across a broad range of settings globally, has been found to be extraordinarily cost-effective.

Eradication is permanent, and so are its benefits, whereas disease control and its costs – mortality, morbidity, and economic – continue into perpetuity. Those children who are at the highest risk of missing out on routine vaccines, including the rural poor, migrants, and nomadic communities, are often at the greatest risk of severe measles disease because of poor nutrition, co-infections, and limited access to health care. Thus, reaching them with measles immunisation can profoundly address health inequalities, particularly when the outreach of services required to reach every child with a measles-containing vaccine can be used as the platform for delivering not only the rubella vaccine – which would result in the concurrent eradication of rubella and congenital rubella syndrome – but other life-saving vaccines as well [60, 61]. Thus, eradication could be considered the ultimate equity mechanism [62].

The Rule of Rescue and the principle of justice leave no ethical excuse if eradication is biologically, technically, operationally, and financially feasible. Smallpox eradication demonstrated that global political will and strong leadership could overcome obstacles and deliver substantial financial savings.

The tools exist to prevent every death from measles and every case of congenital rubella syndrome. Progress could be further accelerated through technological innovations, including microarray patches for vaccine delivery [63].

Countries and partners are accountable for ensuring that all children are protected from these entirely preventable diseases [64]. As measles does not wait, urgent action is required, or each new birth cohort with inadequate immunisation coverage will result in susceptible children accumulating, providing the fuel for the next fiery outbreak [65]. It is time to commit to completing the eradication of measles and rubella viruses so that future generations of children do not live under the shadow of preventable childhood death and disability.

Author details

David N. Durrheim
University of Newcastle, Callaghan, New South Wales, Australia

*Address all correspondence to: david.durrheim@newcastle.edu.au

References

[1] Harper K. Plagues upon the earth. Disease and the course of human history. Princeton: Princeton University Press; 2021. pp. 158–161.

[2] Squire W. On Measles in Fiji. Transactions of the Epidemiological Society of London. 1879;**4**(Pt 1):72–74.

[3] Strebel PM, Cochi SL, Hoekstra E, Rota PA, Featherstone D, Bellini WJ, Katz SL. A world without measles. Journal of Infectious Diseases. 2011;**204** Suppl 1:S1–3. DOI: 10.1093/infdis/jir111.

[4] Orenstein WA, Papania MJ, Wharton ME, Orenstein WA, Papania MJ. 2004. Measles elimination in the United States. Journal of Infectious Diseases. **189**(Suppl 1):S1–3. DOI: 10.1086/377693

[5] Moss WJ, Griffin DE. Measles. Lancet. 2012;**379**:153–164. DOI: 10.1016/S0140-6736(10)62352-5.

[6] Wolfson LJ, Strebel PM, Gacic-Dobo M, Hoekstra EJ, McFarland JW, Hersh BS. Measles initiative. Has the 2005 measles mortality reduction goal been achieved? A natural history modelling study. Lancet. 2007;**369**: 191–200. DOI: 10.1016/S0140-6736(07)60107-X.

[7] Mina MJ, Kula T, Leng Y, Li M, de Vries RD, Knip M, Siljander H, Rewers M, Choy DF, Wilson MS, Larman HB, Nelson AN, Griffin DE, de Swart RL, Elledge SJ. Measles virus infection diminishes preexisting antibodies that offer protection from other pathogens. Science. 2019;**366**:599–606. DOI: 10.1126/science.aay6485.

[8] Shattock AJ, Johnson HC, Sim SY, Carter A, Lambach P, Hutubessy RCW, Thompson KM, Badizadegan K, Lambert B, Ferrari MJ, Jit M, Fu H, Silal SP, Hounsell RA, White RG, Mosser JF, Gaythorpe KAM, Trotter CL, Lindstrand A, O'Brien KL, Bar-Zeev N. Contribution of vaccination to improved survival and health: Modelling 50 years of the expanded programme on immunization. Lancet. 2024;**403**:2307–2316. DOI: 10.1016/S0140-6736.24.00850-X.

[9] Dowdle WR, and Hopkins DR, editors. The eradication of infectious diseases. New York:John Wiley & Sons; 1998. pp. 3–8.

[10] Jenner E. The Origin of the Vaccine Innoculation. London: D.N. Shury; 1801

[11] UNESCO. Records of the smallpox eradication programme of the World Health Organization – memory of the World. 2017. Available from: https://www.unesco.org/en/memory-world/records-smallpox-eradication-programme-world-health-organization. [Accessed: 2025-June-15]

[12] Dowdle WR.The principles of disease elimination and eradication. Bulletin World Health Organisation. 1998;**76**(Suppl 2):22–25

[13] Cochi SL, and Dowdle WR, editors. The eradication of infectious diseases: Understanding the lessons and advancing experience. In Disease Eradication in the 21st Century: Implications for Global Health. online edn. Cambridge, MA: MIT Press Scholarship; 2011. 1–13. DOI: 10.7551/mitpress/9780262016735.003.0001.

[14] Recommendations of the International task force for disease eradication. MMWR Recomm Rep 1993;**42**(RR-16).

[15] Quadros C. Considerations for viral disease eradication: Lessons learned and future strategies: Workshop summary. In: Institute of Medicine (US) Forum on Emerging Infections. National Academies Press; 2002. 22–32. Available at. https://www.ncbi.nlm.nih.gov/books/NBK98114/

[16] Foege WH. House on Fire. The Fight to Eradicate Smallpox. Berkley: University of California Press; 2011

[17] World Health Organization. Proceedings of the Global Technical Consultation to assess the feasibility of measles eradication, 28–30 July 2010. Journal of Infectious Diseases. 2011;**204** (Suppl 1):S4–13. DOI:10.1093/infdis/jir100.

[18] World Health Organization. Meeting of the strategic advisory group of experts on immunization, November 2010. Summary, conclusions and recommendations. Weekly Epidemiological Record. 2011; **86**:1–16

[19] World Health Organization. Global Vaccine Action Plan, 2011–2020. Geneva: World Health Organization; 2013. Available from: http://www.who.int/immunization/global_vaccine_action_plan/en/ [Accessed: 2025-June-15]

[20] Cutts FT, Lessler J, Metcalf CJ. Measles elimination: Progress, challenges and implications for rubella control. Expert Review of Vaccines. 2013;**12**:917–932. DOI: 10.1586/14760584.2013.814847.

[21] Fine PE. Herd immunity: History, theory, practice. Epidemiologic Reviews. 1993;**15**:265–302. DOI: 10.1093/oxfordjournals.epirev.a036121.

[22] Patel MK, Goodson JL, JP Jr A, Kretsinger K, Sodha SV, Steulet C, Gacic-Dobo M, Rota PA, McFarland J, Menning L, Mulders MN, Crowcroft NS. Progress toward regional measles elimination - Worldwide, 2000-2019. MMWR Morbidity and Mortality Weekly Report. 2020;**69**:1700–1705. DOI: 10.15585/mmwr.mm6945a6.

[23] Minta AA, Ferrari M, Antoni S, Portnoy A, Sbarra A, Lambert B, Hatcher C, Hsu CH, Ho LL, Steulet C, Gacic-Dobo M, Rota PA, Mulders MN, Bose AS, Caro WP, O'Connor P, Crowcroft NS. Progress toward measles elimination - Worldwide, 2000-2022. MMWR Morbidity and Mortality Weekly Report. 2023;**72**:1262–1268. DOI: 10.15585/mmwr.mm7246a3.

[24] O'Connor P, Masresha B, Pastor D, Musa N, Hagan J, Khanal S, Lee CW, Crowcroft N. Global Status Report for the verification of measles and rubella elimination, 2022. Vaccines (Basel). 2024;**12**:947. DOI: 10.3390/vaccines12080947.

[25] Durrheim DN, Andrus JK, Tabassum S, Githanga D, Kojouharova M, Talab N. Accelerating global measles and rubella eradication-saving millions of lives, preventing disability, and averting the next pandemic. Vaccines (Basel). 2024;**12**:699. DOI: 10.3390/vaccines12060699.

[26] Durrheim DN, Andrus JK, Tabassum S, Bashour H, Githanga D, Pfaff G. A dangerous measles future looms beyond the COVID-19 pandemic. Nature Medicine. 2021;**27**:360–361. DOI: 10.1038/s41591-021-01237-5.

[27] Durrheim DN, Andrus JK, Tabassum S, Githanga D, Kojouharova M, Teleb N. Global measles eradication goal is urgently needed. Nature. 2025;**641**:1101. DOI: 10.1038/d41586-025-01641-8.

[28] Vynnycky E, Knapp JK, Papadopoulos T, Cutts FT, Hachiya M, Miyano S, Reef SE. Estimates of the global burden of Congenital Rubella Syndrome, 1996-2019. International Journal of Infectious Diseases. 2023;**137**:149–156. DOI: 10.1016/j.ijid.2023.09.003.

[29] Ferrari MJ, Moss WJ. Rubella and measles: The beginning of the endgame. Science. 2025;**388**:32–34. DOI: 10.1126/science.adv7588.

[30] Gastañaduy PA, Banerjee E, DeBolt C, Bravo-Alcántara P, Samad SA, Pastor D, Rota PA, Patel M, Crowcroft NS, Durrheim DN. Public health responses during measles outbreaks in elimination settings: Strategies and challenges. Human Vaccines and Immunotherapeutics. 2018;**14**:2222–2238. DOI: 10.1080/21645515.2018.1474310.

[31] Ortega-Sanchez IR, Vijayaraghavan M, Barskey AE, Wallace GS. The economic burden of sixteen measles outbreaks on United States public health departments in 2011. Vaccine. 2014;**32**:1311–1317. DOI: 10.1016/j.vaccine.2013.10.012.

[32] Dayan GH, Ortega-Sánchez IR, LeBaron CW, Quinlisk MP. Iowa Measles response team. The cost of containing one case of measles: The economic impact on the public health infrastructure–Iowa, 2004. Pediatrics. 2005;**116**:e1–4. DOI: 10.1542/peds.2004-2512.

[33] Thornton J. In the aftermath: The legacy of measles in Samoa. Lancet. 2020;**395**:1535–1536. DOI: 10.1016/S0140-6736(20)31137-5.

[34] Ozawa S, Clark S, Portnoy A, Grewal S, Brenzel L, Walker DG. Return on investment from childhood immunization in low- and middle-income Countries, 2011-20. Health Affairs (Millwood). 2016;**35**:199–207. DOI: 10.1377/hlthaff.2015.1086.

[35] Thompson KM. The health and economic benefits of United States investments in measles and rubella control and elimination. Vaccines (Basel). 2024;**12**:1210. DOI: 10.3390/vaccines12111210.

[36] Thompson KM, Badizadegan ND. Modeling the transmission of measles and rubella to support Global management policy analyses and eradication investment cases. Risk Analysis. 2017;**37**:1109–1131. DOI: 10.1111/risa.12831.

[37] Nelson AM. The cost of disease eradication. Smallpox and Bovine Tuberculosis. Annals of the New York Academy of Sciences. 1999;**894**:83–91. DOI: 10.1111/j.1749-6632.1999.tb08048.x.

[38] UNICEF. Convention on the Rights of the Child; 1999. Available from: http://www.unicef.org/crc. [Accessed: 2025-June-15]

[39] Ryman T, Macauley R, Nshimirimana D, Taylor P, Shimp L, Wilkins K. Reaching every district (RED) approach to strengthen routine immunization services: Evaluation in the African region, 2005. Journal of Public Health. 2010;**32**:18–25. DOI: 10.1038/s41591-021-01237-5.

[40] Hinman AR. Immunization, equity, and human rights. American Journal of Preventive Medicine. 2004;**26**:84–88. DOI: 10.1016/j.amepre.2003.09.008.

[41] Murphy L. Beneficence, law, and liberty: The case of required rescue. Georgetown Law Journal. 2001;**89**: 605–665

[42] McKie J, Richardson J. The rule of rescue. Social Science and Medicine. 2003;**56**:2407–2419. DOI: 10.1016/S0277-9536(02)00244-7.

[43] Jecker NS. The problem with rescue medicine. Journal of Medicine and Philosophy. 2013;**38**:64–81. DOI: 10.1111/risa.12831.

[44] Anderson RM, May RM. Infectious Diseases of humans. dynamics and control. Oxford: Oxford University Press; 1992. p. 70

[45] Levin A, Burgess C, LP Jr G, Bauch C, Babigumira J, Simons E, Dabbagh A. 2011. Global eradication of measles: An epidemiologic and economic evaluation. Journal of Infectious Diseases. **204**(Suppl 1):S98–106. DOI: 10.1093/infdis/jir096

[46] Williams A. Intergenerational equity: An exploration of the 'fair innings' argument. Health Economics. 1997;**6**:117–132. DOI: 10.1002/(sici)1099-1050(199703)6:2.

[47] Durrheim DN, Andrus JK. The ethical case for global measles eradication-justice and the Rule of Rescue. International Health. 2020;**12**:375–377. DOI: 10.1093/inthealth/ihaa038.

[48] Schweitzer A. The Philosophy of Civilization. New York: Prometheus Books; 1987

[49] Andrus JK, de Quadros CA, Solórzano CC, Periago MR, Henderson DA. 2011. Measles and rubella eradication in the Americas. Vaccine. **29** (Suppl 4):D91–96. DOI: 10.1016/j.vaccine.2011.04.059

[50] Durrheim DN, Tuibeqa IV AGS, Grangeon JP, Ogaoga D, Wattiaux A, Mariano KM, Evans R, Hossain S, Aslam SK, Aslam SK. Pacific Island Countries demonstrate the sustained success of a coordinated measles mass vaccination campaign. Lancet Regional Health Western Pacific. 2024;**42**:100998. DOI: 10.1016/j.lanwpc.2023.100998.

[51] Gensler HJ. Ethics and the Golden Rule. Abingdon-on-Thames: Routledge, 2013:84.

[52] World Health Organization. Immunization Agenda 2030. Geneva: World Health Organization; 2020. Available from: https://www.who.int/teams/immunization-vaccines-and-biologicals/strategies/ia2030. [Accessed: 2025-June-15]

[53] Durrheim DN. Measles elimination - using outbreaks to identify and close immunity Gaps. New England Journal of Medicine. 2016;**375**:1392–1393. DOI: 10.1056/NEJMe1610620.

[54] Orenstein WA. The role of measles elimination in development of a national immunization program. Pediatric Infectious Disease Journal. 2006;**25**:1093–1101. DOI: 10.1097/01.inf.0000246840.13477.28.

[55] Fields R, Dabbagh A, Jain M, Sagar KS. 2013. Moving forward with strengthening routine immunization delivery as part of measles and rubella elimination activities. Vaccine. **31**(Suppl 2):B115–21. DOI: 10.1016/j.vaccine.2012.11.094

[56] Hinman AR. Integration of eradication initiatives and health systems. In Cochi SL, and Dowdle WR editors. Disease Eradication in the 21st Century: Implications for Global Health. Cambridge, Massachusetts: MIT Press; 2011. 203–216. 10.7551/mitpress/9186.003.0022.

[57] Caplan AL. Is disease eradication ethical? Lancet. 2009;**373**:2192–2193. DOI: 10.1016/s0140-6736(09)61179-x.

[58] Bayer R. The continuing tensions between individual rights and public health. talking point on public health versus civil liberties. EMBO Reports. 2007;**8**:1099–1103. DOI: 10.1038/sj.embor.7401134.

[59] Bankamp B, Kim G, Hart D, Beck A, Ben Mamou M, Penedos A, Zhang Y, Evans R, Rota PA. Global update on measles molecular epidemiology. Vaccines (Basel). 2024;**12**:810. DOI: 10.3390/vaccines12070810.

[60] Reef SE, Icenogle JP, Plotkin SA. The path to eradication of rubella. Vaccine. 2023;**41**:7525–7531. DOI: 10.1016/j.vaccine.2023.11.014.

[61] Andrus JK, Cochi SL, Cooper LZ, Klein JD. Combining global elimination of measles and rubella with strengthening of health systems in developing Countries. Health Affairs. 2016;**35**:327–333. DOI: 10.1377/hlthaff.2015.1005.

[62] Durrheim DN, Crowcroft NS. The price of delaying measles eradication. Lancet Public Health. 2017;**2**:e130–e131. DOI: 10.1016/S2468-2667(17)30026-9.

[63] Crowcroft NS, Minta AA, Antoni S, Ho LL, Perea W, Mulders MN, Bose AS, Wallace A, Blanc DC, O'Connor PM. Global challenges and solutions to achieving and sustaining measles and rubella elimination. Revista Panamericana de Salud Pública. 2024;**48**:e90. DOI: 10.26633/RPSP.2024.90.

[64] Bachelet M. Data on child deaths are a call for justice. Nature. 2019;**574**:297. DOI: 10.1038/d41586-019-03058-6.

[65] Durrheim DN, Andrus JK, Tabassum S, Githanga D, Kojouharova M, Teleb N. 2025. Measles and rubella eradication: Commitment to a global target is now a matter of urgency. Lancet Infectious Diseases. **25**(7): 716–717. DOI: 10.1016/S1473-3099(25)00307-X

Chapter 3

From a Clinician to an Algorithmic Healer: Navigating the Ethics of Artificial Intelligence in Medical Practice

Abigail Garba and Kudirat Busari

Abstract

Advances in information technology, particularly in the domain of artificial intelligence (AI), have begun to reshape modern society, and medicine is not exempt. In clinical medicine, AI is increasingly integrated into diagnostic processes, risk prediction, treatment planning, robotic-assisted surgery, and administrative workflows. These innovations promise to enhance efficiency and precision, but they also raise complex ethical questions. As healthcare practitioners evolve to adapt to a digitalized landscape, the responsible use of AI must be guided by clear ethical principles to protect both patients and providers. These fundamental ethical principles include autonomy, beneficence, non-maleficence, and justice. Other important guidelines include accountability, transparency, equity, sustainability, and so on. The black box nature of AI models makes transparency challenging, affecting informed consent. Artificial intelligence should improve clinical outcomes without causing undue harm through rigorous validation across diverse clinical contexts. It should not promote automation bias. Additionally, skewed data can lead to data bias; for example, AI trained on data with over 95% of images obtained from white-skinned individuals would perform poorly on dark-skinned individuals. Algorithmic bias may also inadvertently cause AI to perpetuate health disparities. Assigning liability can be complex, creating the need for a shared-accountability approach. Medical education should adapt to foster algorithmic literacy among clinicians. Global policy frameworks and regulatory bodies must evolve alongside technological advances to anticipate new challenges associated with AI. This chapter provides a narrative review of these principles and presents real-world ethical dilemmas that may arise in the everyday clinical application of AI.

Keywords: artificial intelligence, algorithmic healer, ethical principles, medical advances, modern medicine

1. Introduction

Artificial intelligence (AI) is a branch of computer science that enables machines to perform tasks that typically require human intelligence, such as data-driven learning, pattern recognition, understanding languages, and decision-making [1, 2]. It encompasses a range of computational methodologies, including machine learning (ML), deep learning (DL), and natural language processing (NLP), which enable machines to deliver advanced, adaptive, and transformative functions across diverse domains [1–3].

Artificial intelligence is rapidly reshaping the landscape of contemporary medical practice [1, 2]. Due to the exponential growth in computational power, access to vast biomedical datasets, and advances in algorithmic design, AI technologies now demonstrate the ability to outperform human clinicians in specific tasks such as image recognition and predictive analytics [2–4]. These systems can assimilate heterogeneous data, including electronic health records, genomic data, imaging studies, and wearable device outputs, to uncover complex non-linear patterns that are often imperceptible to the human eye [1, 4, 5]. Consequently, AI is being integrated into a wide array of clinical domains, including diagnostics, treatment planning, risk stratification, prognostication, and real-time patient monitoring [1, 4, 5].

Although the term "algorithmic healer" is not yet standardized in medical literature, it is understood to refer to a clinician whose capacity to diagnose, prognosticate, and treat patients is substantially enhanced through collaboration with algorithmic systems, especially AI-driven tools, while retaining ultimate responsibility and oversight. This concept reflects the fact that AI augments human judgment rather than substituting for it, and the clinician remains responsible for validation, contextual interpretation, and ethical decision-making [6].

The paradigm shift is not merely technological, as it also carries profound ethical implications [7, 8]. The introduction of algorithmically mediated decision-making into clinical care challenges foundational concepts of medical ethics and professional responsibilities [1, 7, 8]. As we transition from traditional clinician-centered care to AI-augmented care, critical ethical questions emerge [7–10]:

- How do we ensure informed patient consent and safeguard autonomy in AI-augmented care?
- What level of transparency is required for building and maintaining trust while utilizing algorithmic tools?
- How do we detect and mitigate inherent algorithmic biases that can lead to discriminatory outcomes?
- Who would ultimately be accountable when AI systems contribute to diagnostic or therapeutic errors?
- And, most importantly, what will be the evolving role of the human clinician in the era of digital augmentation?

This chapter seeks to explore these issues in depth. It aims to provide a balanced perspective on how traditional medical ethical principles can be upheld and strengthened as AI advances in medicine, ensuring that human dignity is protected while harnessing AI's transformative benefits.

2. Historical context and evolution of artificial intelligence in medicine

Artificial intelligence emerged as a formal discipline in the mid 1950s during the Dartmouth Conference, where John McCarthy coined the term. Earlier developments, including Christopher Strachey's 1951 AI program, marked the nascent phase of AI as a primarily academic endeavor [1]. Its application in medicine has evolved significantly over the past decades, paralleling broader advances in computer science and data availability. Early milestones relevant to healthcare began with the development of rule-based expert systems in the 1970s and 1980s [1, 5]. One of the most notable examples was MYCIN, an early AI program designed to diagnose and recommend treatment for severe bacterial infections by utilizing a knowledge base of if–then rules to mimic clinical reasoning; this was a foundational step in the integration of AI into medical decision-making [11, 12].

The early systems were limited by their reliance on explicitly programmed logic, which proved inflexible and difficult to scale across diverse clinical scenarios [1, 11]. A pivotal advancement in the evolution of AI was the emergence of ML, which transitioned the field from rule-based systems to data-driven models. Machine-learning algorithms are designed to identify patterns and optimize performance through iterative learning from empirical data, without the need for task-specific programming [1, 11, 13]. This progress was further accelerated by the development of DL, a specialized branch of ML that employs the use of multi-layered artificial neural networks to extract hierarchical features from large-scale, multi-dimensional datasets. DL has been instrumental in achieving state-of-the-art performance in complex domains such as medical image analysis, NLP, and speech recognition [8, 11, 13]. **Figures 1** and **2** depict the natural evolution of AI since its inception and the relationship between various sub-fields of AI.

The incorporation of AI technologies into healthcare has led to significant advancements across several domains. In diagnostics, AI algorithms demonstrate expert-level accuracy in interpreting radiological images, including X-rays, mammograms, and computed tomography scans [14]. Similarly,DL models are now used in identifying skin lesions and differentiating between benign and malignant lesions [14, 15]. Furthermore, the Food and Drug Administration (FDA) has approved three AI devices as autonomous screening tools for diabetic retinopathy (DR), including the EyeArt, A Eye health and IDx-DR AI systems. These systems have a sensitivity and specificity of greater than 87% and 90%, respectively, for the early detection of more-than-mild DR, necessitating referral to ophthalmologists for intervention [16]. In treatment planning, AI tools assist in individualizing therapeutic regimens by analyzing patient-specific data and evidence-based guidelines [17]. AI is also increasingly transforming pharmaceutical research with the advent of "digital twins," which act as virtual replicas of biological systems or patient-specific profiles. These models allow researchers to simulate drug discovery, formulation, design, and

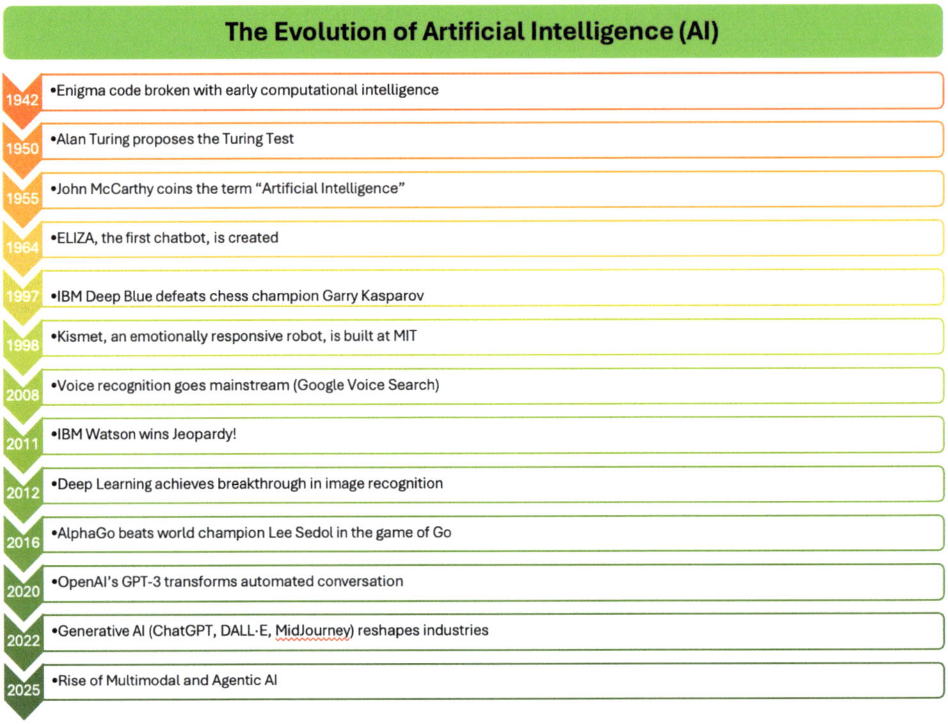

Figure 1.
The evolution of artificial intelligence.

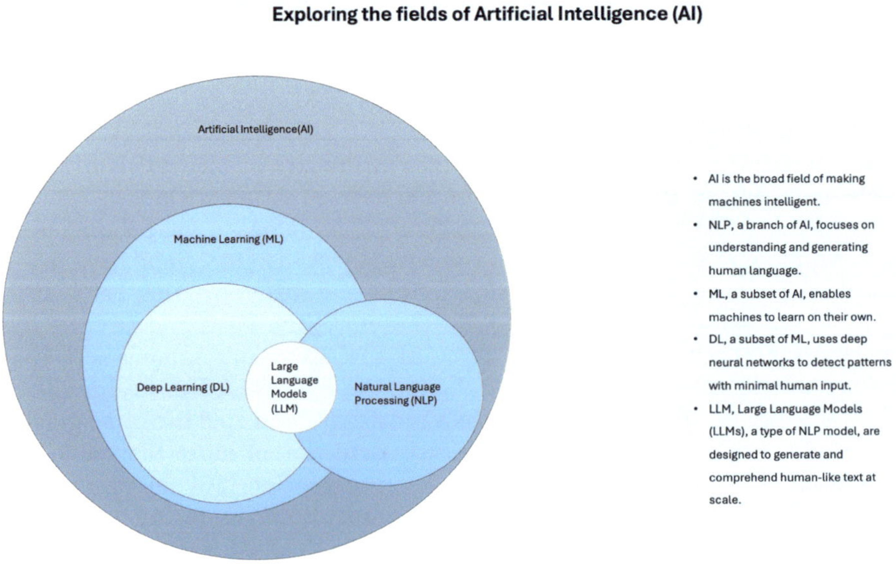

Figure 2.
Exploring the fields of artificial intelligence.

efficacy testing *in silico*, thereby reducing reliance on costly and time-consuming *in vivo* or clinical trials [18].

Predictive analytics leverages AI to anticipate disease progression, hospital readmissions, and clinical deterioration, thereby enabling timely and preventive care [17]. Natural language processing enables the extraction and interpretation of structured information from unstructured clinical narratives [19]. This facilitates automated summarization of patient notes, identification of risk factors, and support for clinical coding and documentation [19]. More recently, the advent of large language models (LLMs), such as OpenAI's GPT-4 and Google's Med-PaLM, has extended AI's capabilities to clinical reasoning, answering medical questions, and providing clinical decision support [19]. While promising, these tools raise concerns about factual accuracy.

The evolution from early symbolic rule-based systems to contemporary deep neural architectures has improved the accuracy and efficiency of clinical decision-making while simultaneously raising concerns regarding algorithmic transparency, interpretability, and seamless integration into clinical practice [1, 9, 13]. **Tables 1** and 2 depict the current applications of AI in healthcare.

3. Ethical principles in the era of artificial intelligence

The use of AI in medicine must be governed by the fundamental ethical principles of biomedical practice, which include autonomy, beneficence, non-maleficence, and justice. These principles remain central to ethically sound clinical decision-making and must be interpreted in the context of algorithmic systems [7, 20]. Other important guidelines governing the use of AI in healthcare include accountability and responsibility, transparency and explainability, inclusivity and equity, privacy, trust, sustainability, dignity, and solidarity [21, 22].

- ***Respect for Autonomy:*** This entails a patient's right to informed decision-making regarding their care. In the context of AI, this requires transparency regarding how algorithmic models contribute to clinical decisions and the extent to which they influence diagnoses, risk predictions, or therapeutic plans [20, 22]. Given the complexity and often opaque "black box" nature of many AI models, especially DL and LLMs, meaningful transparency becomes a challenge [22]. Patients may struggle to comprehend how or why an AI system has arrived at a particular recommendation, yet, informed consent requires that they be aware of the roles these systems play. Thus, explainability and interpretability are not merely technical requirements but ethical imperatives necessary to uphold patient autonomy [20, 22].

- ***Beneficence and non-maleficence:*** These principles compel clinicians and developers to ensure that AI applications in healthcare demonstrably improve clinical outcomes without causing undue harm [7, 20]. This involves rigorous validation of AI systems across diverse populations and clinical contexts prior to deployment. High-stakes settings such as emergency medicine, oncology, and intensive care units pose risks, where erroneous predictions or over-reliance on unvalidated tools can result in

Applications of Artificial Intelligence in Healthcare Delivery	
Diagnosis	Interpretation of medical images in radiology, pathology, and dermatology.
	Interpretation of laboratory results
	Clinical decision support, e.g., Babylon Health, Isabel, DXplain.
	Genomics and precision diagnostics, e.g., identifying mutations or biomarkers for specific diseases.
	Detection of arrhythmias, ischemia, early heart disease
	Direct-to-consumer applications
Prevention	Estimating risk of chronic disease
	Detection of outbreaks
	Personalized recommendations for diet, exercise, and medication adherence.
	Identification of high-risk patients before clinical deterioration.
	Interpretation of genetic data to recommend preventive interventions.
Treatment	Drug delivery systems optimization
	Evidence-based decision-making and treatment plans
	Precision therapy–tailored treatments based on genomic, clinical, and lifestyle data
	Robotic surgery and procedural assistance, e.g., the da Vinci Surgical System.
	Remote patient monitoring, e.g., wearables for monitoring glucose for AI-guided insulin therapy.
	Use of chatbots and apps in mental health and behavioral therapy, e.g., Woebot, Tess.
	Robotic health companions, such as socially assistive robots, healthcare and monitoring robots, cognitive and emotional support robots, and telepresence robots.
	"Uberization" of healthcare – On-demand, app-driven delivery of services, e.g., virtual consultations, home care, and transportation.
Administration	Speech-to-text transcription of clinical encounters
	Automated summaries, e.g., of visits, results, and discharge summaries.
	Appointment scheduling
	Optimizing resource allocation, e.g., the use of imaging, rooms, beds, and staff.
	Automated billing and coding
	Streamlining patient communication, e.g., chatbots for prescription refills and test preparation instructions.
	Automated triage systems
	Multilingual patient interaction support
	Inventory management
	Referrals management
	Data management and reporting

Table 1.
Examples of AI applications in healthcare delivery.

catastrophic consequences [7]. Additionally, non-maleficence implies that the introduction of AI should not degrade doctor–patient relationships, diminish clinical reasoning, or promote "automation bias". Automation bias

Applications of Artificial Intelligence in Medical Research and Education	
Clinical research	Patient recruitment and eligibility matching
	Predictive modeling e.g., predicting dropout risk.
	Trial design optimization
	Monitoring and safety
	Data extraction and cleaning
	Reduction of operational costs, e.g., by streamlining administrative tasks.
	Analysis of laboratory and clinical data
	Patient engagement and retention, e.g., improving adherence to protocols using chatbots.
Pharmacology	Drug discovery e.g. Atomwise
	Prediction of pharmacokinetics
	Prediction of pharmacodynamics
	Digital twins in drug efficacy studies
	Drug repurposing
	Adverse drug reaction prediction
	Precision medicine – tailoring drug selection and dosing based on genetics, biomarkers, and patient data
Medical education	Adaptive learning platforms e.g. Lecturio
	Virtual patients and simulations
	Intelligent tutoring systems that provide real-time feedback on case-based exercises.
	Assessment and analytics, e.g., automated scoring of assessment responses.
	Use of natural language processing, e.g., personalized reading lists and extraction of information from medical literature.
	Medical imaging training in radiology, pathology, dermatology, and cardiology.
	Virtual reality and augmented reality integration, e.g., to enhance anatomy teaching and surgical skills acquisition.

Table 2.
Examples of AI applications in medical research and education.

is a phenomenon where human decision-makers overly trust algorithmic outputs despite contrary evidence.

- ***Justice:*** This principle emphasizes the fair distribution of healthcare resources and the avoidance of discrimination [20, 22]. In the AI context, this translates into ensuring equity in both the design and application of algorithmic tools. It also demands that AI systems do not exacerbate existing disparities in healthcare access [22, 23]. Several empirical studies have documented embedded biases in AI systems trained on skewed datasets, resulting in racial, gender, or socio-economic disparities in clinical predictions, such as the underestimation of illness severity in Black patients or differential access to diagnostics [10, 22]. Algorithmic fairness, therefore, requires inclusive and representative training datasets as well as active auditing for disparate impacts across sub-populations. In addition, the concept of justice also involves addressing the "digital divide", as under-resourced healthcare systems may lack the infrastructure to deploy or benefit from AI tools, thereby risking the amplification of global health inequities [10, 20, 22, 23].

- ***Accountability:*** This, in AI-assisted healthcare, presents complex ethical and legal challenges. In traditional medicine, responsibility is assigned to the clinician, who is expected to exercise professional judgment and uphold the duty of care. However, with AI influencing diagnosis and therapy, assigning liability becomes less straightforward. When harm results from AI-assisted decisions, questions arise about whether the blame lies with the clinician, the AI developer, the institution, or regulatory bodies [7, 22]. This ambiguity may discourage clinicians from fully integrating AI into practice without clear legal frameworks [22, 24]. A shared accountability approach is increasingly advocated to surmount this challenge. Developers must ensure algorithmic validity, transparency, and fairness; institutions must implement robust oversight mechanisms; and clinicians must understand AI limitations and remain the ultimate decision-makers [24]. Explainability tools are also essential to enable traceability and maintain ethical standards. As AI systems become more autonomous, developing clear guidelines and legal structures will be critical for ensuring patient safety and upholding trust in AI-enhanced care [22, 24].

4. Blurring the line of human–machine collaboration: The role of the clinician in the age of artificial intelligence

As AI becomes more widely incorporated into clinical workflows, its role is increasingly understood as a tool for augmentation rather than a replacement for physicians. Artificial intelligence systems can support clinicians by enhancing diagnostic accuracy, streamlining administrative tasks, and reducing cognitive workload [7, 14]. Nevertheless, the clinician remains central in synthesizing AI outputs with the nuanced realities of individual patient care, considering biomedical, psychosocial, cultural, and emotional contexts. Interpreting algorithmic recommendations through a human lens ensures that clinical decisions remain patient-centric, ethically sound, and contextually appropriate [22, 25, 26].

Beyond the analytical capacity, the physician's unique ability to convey empathy, build trust, and offer reassurance remains irreplaceable. Algorithms lack the capacity for compassion, moral reasoning, and interpersonal relationships, all of which are crucial elements, particularly when patients face uncertainties, fears, or suffering [25, 26]. It is noteworthy, however, that the increasing reliance on AI introduces potential risks such as "automation complacency" or automation bias, where clinicians accept algorithmic outputs without question, and trust miscalibration, where either over-reliance or undue skepticism of AI impairs clinical judgment [20, 22, 26].

To mitigate these risks, the concept of "clinical override" has been proposed, whereby clinicians intentionally diverge from AI recommendations, and this must be preserved and supported at all times. In addition, medical education must adapt to foster "algorithmic literacy", ensuring clinicians understand AI's capabilities, limitations, and ethical implications. This dual emphasis on

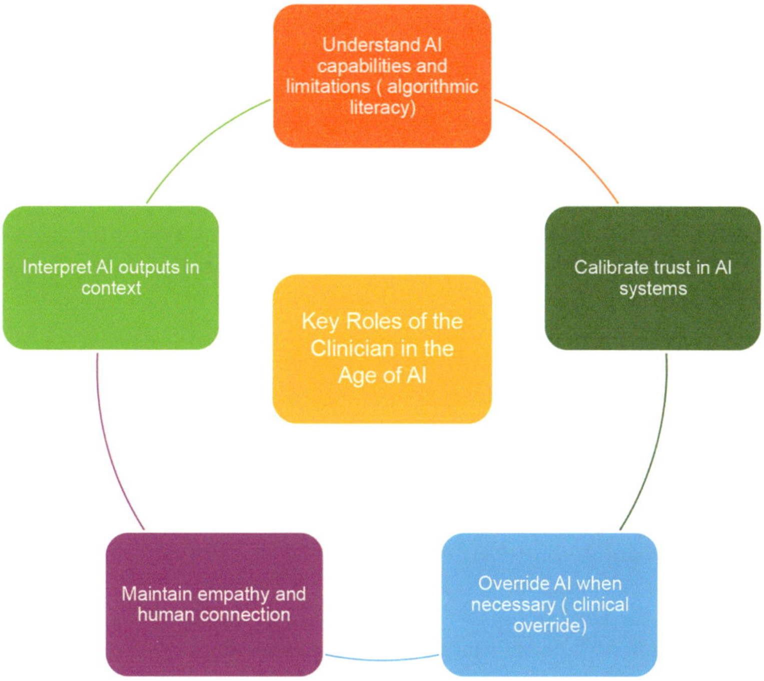

Figure 3.
Key roles of the clinician in the age of artificial intelligence.

humanism and technological fluency is critical for the safe, effective, and equitable integration of AI into modern medical practices [22, 25, 26]. **Figure 3** is a schematic diagram summarizing the key roles of the clinician in the era of AI.

5. Informed consent and data ethics

Integrating AI into clinical workflows presents significant ethical challenges, particularly concerning informed consent and data stewardship [7, 22]. Conventional informed consent processes are grounded in the principle of patient autonomy, which assumes that patients can understand and evaluate the potential risks and benefits of medical interventions [22, 24, 27]. However, the use of AI complicates this process, as many advanced models, especially those built on DL and LLMs, operate as "black boxes" whose decision-making processes are not readily explainable, even by experts [22, 27]. This opacity presents significant challenges to clinicians in explaining AI-generated recommendations to patients in a way that enables truely informed decision-making [22, 25].

In parallel, the use of AI in healthcare relies heavily on large volumes of patient data collated from electronic health records, genetic data, and wearable devices [4]. This shift toward continuous health data acquisition prompts critical concerns regarding the ownership, usage, governance, and safeguarding of personal health information [17, 22]. Although data is vital for developing effective AI models, ethical issues arise over whether patients are adequately informed about the purposes, sharing practices, and potential commercialization of their health information [17, 22, 24]. Furthermore, in the era of ubiquitous surveillance and ongoing data harvesting, consent is no longer a one-time event but a continuous process [7, 22, 28]. Patients are often unaware that their physiological metrics, behavioral data, and social determinants are passively captured through wearable technologies and digital health systems [20, 22, 28]. This warrants the development of dynamic consent models that enable individuals to modify their data-sharing preferences over time, thereby maintaining personal agency [29]. Ethical AI implementation must therefore prioritize transparency, accountability, and robust data governance mechanisms that protect patient privacy while fostering responsible innovation [22, 29].

6. Bias and algorithmic inequality

Bias is a prejudice or unfairness that may be introduced even before AI starts being used in a clinical setting. If AI is trained on a dataset obtained from imbalanced population data, that AI will always perform in a manner that negatively affects under-represented groups [30]. Bias in AI systems is usually a reflection of patterns of discrimination that are present in most other areas of life, thus affecting social justice, equality, and even trust in technology at large [30]. Two essential kinds of bias related to AI systems are data bias and algorithmic bias [30].

Example 1:
A neural network in Heidelberg was trained to differentiate malignant and benign melanomas from clinical images. It was trained on over 100,000 photographs and was found to outperform 58 dermatologists across 17 countries. However, over 95 percent of the images it was trained on were obtained from white-skinned individuals, which could cause it to perform poorly on dark-skinned individuals [31]. This aligns with research findings that biased training datasets result in biased diagnostic performances of AI [32].

Example 2:
An algorithm was designed to identify patients with complex health needs based on healthcare costs so that health systems could provide extra support [10]. This was based on the assumption that sicker patients have higher healthcare costs. However, Black patients with the same level of illness as White patients had lower healthcare costs than their counterparts due to unequal access to care. This led to the algorithm systematically underestimating the needs of Black patients, with the algorithm identifying only 17.7% of Black patients as needing extra support, whereas correcting for the bias would have increased that percentage to 46.5%. Despite its presumed accuracy, this algorithmic bias caused AI to perpetuate inequities and limit support for a vulnerable group.

Ethical and practical strategies to audit and mitigate bias include [30, 33, 34]:

- Diversifying training datasets
- Dataset augmentation or reweighting

- Transparency in decision-making by AI systems.
- Regular audits of AI performance conducted by institutions.
- Collaboration among developers, ethicists, clinicians, and patients for the development of AI systems.
- Standardization of all AI models should include processes for diversity and inclusion.
- Regular training of clinicians on the use of AI systems and their biases is essential.
- Regular reports by clinicians on how AI diagnostic systems perform with different populations help AI developers improve quality.
- Research and development of new AI systems with due ethical considerations.

7. Legal, regulatory, and policy considerations

The regulatory landscape governing the integration of AI in healthcare is rapidly evolving but remains complex and heterogeneous across different jurisdictions [18]. In the European Union (EU), the proposed Artificial Intelligence Act adopts a risk-based stratification for AI systems, designating most medical AI applications as "high-risk" [35]. This classification mandates stringent safeguards, including rigorous pre-deployment testing, transparency requirements, human oversight provisions, and continuous post-marketing surveillance to ensure safety and reliability [35]. In contrast, regulatory oversight in the United States is guided primarily by the FDA Software as a Medical Device (SaMD) framework. This framework focuses on lifecycle regulation and the need to mitigate risks such as "algorithmic drift", which refers to the decline in AI model performance as clinical contexts and datasets evolve over time [36, 37]. Other legal and regulatory frameworks that have been developed in various parts of the world are summarized in **Table 3** below. These differing jurisdictional approaches reflect the broader challenge of balancing innovation with patient safety in an AI-enabled healthcare environment [18].

Compliance with data protection frameworks, such as the General Data Protection Regulation (GDPR) in Europe and the Health Insurance Portability and Accountability Act (HIPAA) in the United States, remains a cornerstone of trustworthy AI deployment [7, 18, 21]. These frameworks establish the standards for the lawful collection, processing, and safeguarding of patient data [7, 18, 21].

The issue of liability and the traceability of harm in AI-augmented clinical practice introduces an additional layer of complexity [21]. Traditional malpractice laws hold clinicians accountable when medical care falls below accepted professional standards. However, assigning responsibility in AI-assisted healthcare is challenging due to the involvement of multiple stakeholders, raising both legal and ethical concerns [7, 21, 22]. Experts debate whether clinicians should be regarded as the final decision-makers, whether AI developers should bear part of the liability, or whether healthcare institutions should share responsibility. This diffusion of accountability can result in inadequate

Country	Year	Regulatory Organization	Title of Policy Document
United Kingdom	2019	National Institute for Health and Care Excellence – National Health Services	Evidence Standards Framework for Digital Health Technologies
	2021	Medicines and Healthcare Products Regulatory Agency	Software and AI as a Medical Device Change Program
	2022	The Regulatory Horizons Council	The Regulation of AI as a Medical Device
Australia	2019	The Royal Australian and New Zealand College of Radiologists	Ethical Principles for AI in Medicine
	2021	Therapeutic Goods (Medical Devices) Regulation	Regulatory Changes for Software-Based Medical Devices
Brazil	2021	Brazilian Chamber of Deputies	The Brazilian Legal Framework for AI
China	2019	National Medical Products Administration	Technical Guideline on AI-aided Software
	2021	National Medical Products Administration	Guidelines for the Classification and Definition of Artificial Intelligence-Based Software as a Medical Device
	2022	The Centre for Medical Device Evaluation	Guidelines for Registration and Review of Artificial Intelligence-Based Medical Devices
Singapore	2021	Singapore Ministry of Health	AI in Healthcare Guidelines
	2022	Health Sciences Authority	Regulatory Guidelines for SaMD: A Lifecycle Approach

Table 3.
Legal and regulatory frameworks for healthcare artificial intelligence in different countries.

compensation for harmed individuals, incomplete recognition or remediation of harm, and erosion of public trust in AI technologies [21]. Additionally, in some cases, clinicians also run the risk of becoming "liability sinks" that disproportionately absorb the blame for adverse outcomes resulting from AI-based clinical decisions. To mitigate this, "shared accountability frameworks" outline how AI developers should ensure algorithmic validity and fairness, healthcare institutions should provide implementation governance and training, and clinicians should exercise critical judgment to override AI outputs when clinically warranted [18, 22].

At the global level, ethical and regulatory guidance continues to emerge. The World Health Organization (WHO) 2021 Guidance on Ethics and Governance of Artificial Intelligence for Health provides a normative framework emphasizing respect for human rights, transparency, equity, and stakeholder accountability throughout the AI lifecycle [38, 39]. Complementary efforts include the collaboration between the International Telecommunication Union and WHO to form the Focus Group on AI for Health (FG-AI4H). This focus group developed benchmarking protocols to evaluate AI systems for safety, accuracy, and clinical efficacy across several domains [39]. Furthermore, the United Nations Educational, Scientific and Cultural Organization's 2021 Recommendation on the Ethics of Artificial Intelligence has been adopted by over sixty countries. It articulates foundational principles centered around human dignity, fairness, inclusivity, and sustainability, thereby serving as an ethical anchor for global AI governance [40].

Collectively, these frameworks and evolving regulatory models underscore the need for adaptive governance that can balance regulatory rigor with innovation and global harmonization across all sectors. Establishing clear mechanisms of accountability, robust data protection, and ethical oversight will be essential as AI becomes increasingly integral to healthcare delivery [7, 21].

8. Looking forward: Ethics by design

As AI continues to advance, new ethical frontiers emerge beyond those already described in current clinical practice. The emergence of generative AI and LLMs raises profound questions about intellectual ownership, authorship, accountability for AI-generated content, and the potential dissemination of misinformation within clinical and public health domains [7, 22, 41]. These technologies also reshape patient–provider dynamics, as conversational agents and decision-support systems increasingly influence how patients access and interpret medical information. Therefore, ensuring accuracy, minimizing bias, and preserving trust in clinical expertise remain crucial [21, 22, 41].

Innovations such as synthetic data and digital twins provide promising avenues for accelerating biomedical research, enabling predictive modeling and advancing personalized medicine [7, 18]. However, their adoption raises concerns about the fidelity and representativeness of simulated data, the risk of perpetuating systemic biases, and potential misuse in contexts beyond their intended scope. These issues underscore the need for rigorous validation processes, transparent reporting standards, and strong ethical safeguards to ensure responsible deployment.

Looking ahead, global policy frameworks must also evolve in tandem with these technological advances. Regulatory bodies will need to anticipate novel challenges posed by generative AI, especially in domains such as authorship attribution, intellectual property rights, and cross-border data flows [18, 22, 23, 41].

Equally important is equipping the next generation of clinicians for AI-integrated practice. Medical education must undergo a paradigm shift to include competencies in digital literacy, algorithmic ethics, data stewardship, and critical appraisal of AI tools [42]. Training clinicians not only to utilize but to question and contextualize AI outputs will be vital to maintaining clinical autonomy, preventing automation bias, and ensuring that human judgment and empathy remain central to patient care [7, 22]. Integrating these elements into medical curricula and continuous professional development will produce clinicians skilled at harnessing AI's potential while upholding ethical and professional standards [42].

9. Real-world ethical dilemmas arising from the use of artificial intelligence in clinical settings

The following scenarios highlight how AI can improve accuracy, efficiency, and scalability in medicine, while also raising ethical challenges related to bias, accountability, transparency, privacy, and fairness.

Scenario 1

When AI is used to identify high-risk patients for extra monitoring or resources, could it underestimate the needs and risks of a vulnerable group due to systemic barriers to care, and could this lead to inequitable resource allocation?

This scenario challenges the principles of justice (care may be distributed unfairly) and non-maleficence (patients may be harmed through under-treatment).

Scenario 2

When DL models are used to diagnose without the reasoning being clear—for example, in cases of diabetic retinopathy – do clinicians feel pressured to trust "black box" outputs, even when they are unsure of how decisions are made? This scenario challenges the principles of autonomy (patients may be unable to make informed choices without understanding how decisions are made), beneficence (clinicians may struggle to use AI to act in the patient's best interest), and non-maleficence (patients may be harmed by errors that cannot be questioned or explained).

Scenario 3

When hospitals partner with tech companies to train AI using large sets of de-identified patient data, patients are not explicitly asked for consent. Is re-identification of patients possible through cross-referencing? This scenario challenges the principles of autonomy (patients may lose control over their personal health data) and justice (marginalized groups may be disproportionately harmed if their data is misused or inadequately protected).

Scenario 4

When AI tools outperform humans, for example, in detecting lung nodules or breast cancer on imaging, should AI results override a radiologist's interpretation? If there is a conflict, who is accountable and liable for a missed diagnosis or medical error – the clinician, the hospital, or the AI developer? This scenario challenges the principles of beneficence (the duty to act in the patient's best interest may be outsourced to AI), non-maleficence (there may be a risk of harm from unquestioned reliance on AI), and justice (responsibility not being fairly assigned).

Scenario 5

When AI-driven tools are more available and accessible in resource-rich hospitals and countries, underserved communities are left behind. This scenario challenges the principles of justice (as benefits may be distributed unfairly) and beneficence (the duty to improve health broadly rather than reinforcing privilege).

Scenario 6

When AI chatbots are used in mental health – for example, to screen for depression or provide basic therapy support – patients may disclose suicidal ideation. Who is responsible for timely intervention: the AI developer, the clinician, or the health system? This scenario challenges the principles of autonomy (individuals may not fully understand they are engaging with a machine, limiting their ability to make an informed choice), beneficence (chatbots may improve access to care), non-maleficence (poorly designed or inadequately supervised chatbots may give harmful advice, miss warning signs of suicidality, or fail to escalate emergencies appropriately), and justice (expanding access to underserved populations while potentially providing less effective care to marginalized communities, for example, due to language barriers).

DOI: http://dx.doi.org/10.5772/intechopen.1012764

Scenario 7

When AI models predict which patients are most likely to benefit from scarce resources like ventilators or donor organs, could AI embed biases against vulnerable groups (e.g., against people with disabilities or marginalized communities), thereby skewing who receives life-saving treatment? This scenario challenges the principles of justice (fair distribution of life-saving care *versus* reinforcing existing health inequities), autonomy (patients and families having little understanding of how these critical choices are made), beneficence (maximizing overall health benefit *versus* prioritizing those most likely to recover), and non-maleficence (preventable harm caused by denying care to patients who could have benefited). It also highlights the difficult balance between justice for the population and beneficence toward the individual patient.

10. Conclusion

The integration of AI into medicine offers unprecedented opportunities for advancing diagnostics, therapeutics, and healthcare delivery while simultaneously raising complex ethical and governance challenges. Anchoring AI deployment in ethical principles and guidelines ensures that the transition from clinician to algorithmic healer enhances, rather than undermines, the ethical foundations of medical practice. Respect for patient autonomy involves prioritizing transparency, accountability, and data governance. To ensure beneficence and patient safety, explainability tools should be integrated into AI applications to enable traceability and uphold trust in AI-enhanced care. Non-maleficence implies that the introduction of AI should not degrade doctor–patient relationships. Clinical override may be required, permitting clinicians to intentionally diverge from AI recommendations to avoid harm to the patient. Inclusive and representative training datasets would ensure algorithmic fairness, and addressing the digital divide would improve access in disadvantaged healthcare systems, thus ensuring justice for all. As clinical practice stands at the intersection of innovation and tradition, the task ahead is to foster a synergistic model in which humans and machines collaborate to provide safe and equitable healthcare without becoming competing agents.

Acknowledgments

The authors acknowledge Aishah Busari for preparing the figures and graphical illustrations.

The authors acknowledge the use of ChatGPT (OpenAI, San Francisco, CA, USA) for assistance with the initial generation of concepts and grammar refinement. All AI-generated suggestions were critically reviewed, refined, and developed by the authors, who take full responsibility for the final content.

Conflict of interest

The authors have no conflicts of interest to declare.

Author details

Abigail Garba[1*] and Kudirat Busari[2]

1 University of Alberta, Edmonton, Canada

2 Zenith Medical and Kidney Centre, Abuja, Nigeria

*Address all correspondence to: theonlygail@gmail.com

References

[1] Alowais SA, Alghamdi SS, Alsuhebany N, Alqahtani T, Alshaya AI, Almohareb SN, et al. Revolutionizing healthcare: The role of artificial intelligence in clinical practice. BMC Medical Education. 2023;**23**:689

[2] Khosravi M, Mojtabaeian SM, Demiray EKD, Sayar B. A systematic review of the outcomes of utilization of artificial intelligence within the healthcare systems of the Middle East: A thematic analysis of findings. Health Science Reports. 2024;**7** (12):e70300

[3] Qi Y, Mohamad E, Azlan AA, Zhang C. Utilization of artificial intelligence in clinical practice: A systematic review of China's experiences. Digit Health. 2025;**11**:1–21

[4] Obermeyer Z, Emanuel EJ. Predicting the future—big data, machine learning, and clinical medicine. New England Journal of Medicine. 2016;**375**(13):1216

[5] Jiang F, Jiang Y, Zhi H, Dong Y, Li H, Ma S, et al. Artificial intelligence in healthcare: Past, present and future. Stroke and Vascular Neurology. 2017;**2**(4):230–243

[6] Panahi O. The algorithmic healer: AI's impact on public health delivery. Journal of Medical Case Reports. 2025;**3** (1):759–762

[7] Gerke S, Minssen T, Cohen G. Ethical legal challenges of artificial intelligence-driven healthcare. In: Bohr A, and Memarzadeh K, editors. Artificial Intelligence in Healthcare. 1st ed. Cambridge, MA: Elsevier; 2020. p. 295–336

[8] Aravazhi PS, Gunasekaran P, Benjamin NZY, Thai A, Chandrasekar KK, Kolanu ND, et al. The integration of artificial intelligence into clinical medicine: Trends, challenges, and future directions. Disease-a-Month. 2025;**71**(6):101882

[9] Park CW, Seo SW, Kang N, Ko B, Choi BW, Park CM, et al. Artificial intelligence in health care: Current applications and issues. The Journal of Korean Medical Science 2020;**35**:1–11

[10] Obermeyer Z, Powers B, Vogeli C, Mullainathan S. Dissecting racial bias in an algorithm used to manage the health of populations. Science. 2019;**366** (6464):447–453

[11] Yu KH, Beam AL, Kohane IS. Artificial intelligence in healthcare. Nature Biomedical Engineering. 2018;**2** (10):719–731

[12] Shortliffe EH. Computer-based Medical Consultations: MYCIN. 2nd ed. New York: Elsevier; 2012. p. 239

[13] Nguyen TT, Larrivée N, Lee A, Bilaniuk O, Durand R.Use of artificial intelligence in dentistry: Current clinical trends and research advances. The Journal of the Canadian Dental Association. 2021;**87**(l7):1488–2159

[14] Najjar R. Redefining radiology: A review of artificial intelligence integration in medical imaging. Diagnostics. 2023;**13**(17):2760

[15] Esteva A, Kuprel B, Novoa RA, Ko J, Swetter SM, Blau HM, et al. Dermatologist-level classification of skin cancer with deep neural networks. Nature 2017;**542**:115–118

[16] Alqahtani AS, Alshareef WM, Aljadani HT, Hawsawi WO, Shaheen MH. The efficacy of artificial intelligence in diabetic retinopathy screening: A systematic review and meta-analysis. International Journal of Retina and Vitreous. 2025;**11**(1):48

[17] Rajkomar A, Oren E, Chen K, Dai AM, Hajaj N, Hardt M, et al. Scalable and accurate deep learning with electronic health records. Npj Digital Medicine. 2018;**1**:18

[18] Palaniappan K, Lin EYT, Vogel S. Global regulatory frameworks for the use of artificial intelligence (AI) in the healthcare services sector. Healthcare. 2024;**12**(5):562

[19] Paulraj NJ.Natural language processing on clinical notes: Advanced techniques for risk prediction and summarization. Journal of Computer Science and Technology Studies. 2025;**7**(3):494–502

[20] Floridi L, Cowls J, Beltrametti M, Chatila R, Chazerand P, Dignum V, et al. AI4People—An ethical framework for a good AI society: Opportunities, risks, principles, and recommendations. Minds and Machines 2018;**28**:689–707

[21] Mennella C, Maniscalco U, De Pietro G, Esposito M. Ethical and regulatory challenges of AI technologies in healthcare: A narrative review. Heliyon. 2024;**10**(4):1-20

[22] Jha D, Durak G, Sharma V, Keles E, Cicek V, Zhang Z, et al. A conceptual framework for applying ethical principles of AI to medical practice. Bioengineering 2025;**12**:180

[23] Jobin A, Ienca M, Vayena E. The global landscape of AI ethics guidelines. Nature Machine Intelligence. 2019;**1**(9):389–399

[24] Morley J, Machado CCV, Burr C, Cowls J, Joshi I, Taddeo M, et al.. The ethics of AI in health care: A mapping review. Social Science & Medicine. 2020;**260**:1–14

[25] Jotterand F, Bosco C. Keeping the "human in the loop" in the age of artificial intelligence: Accompanying commentary for "correcting the brain?" by Rainey and Erden. Science and Engineering Ethics. 2020;**26**(5):2455–2460

[26] Jotterand F, Bosco C. Artificial intelligence in medicine: A sword of damocles?. Journal of Medical Systems. 2022;**46**(1):9

[27] Andreotta AJ, Kirkham N, Rizzi M. AI, big data, and the future of consent. AI and Society. 2022;**37**(4):1715–1728

[28] Mittelstadt B. From individual to group privacy in big data analytics. Philosophy and Technology. 2017;**30**(4):475–494

[29] Kotsenas AL, Balthazar P, Andrews D, Geis JR, Cook TS. Rethinking patient consent in the era of artificial intelligence and big data. Journal of the American College of Radiology. 2021;**18**(1):180–184

[30] Owolabi OO, Adewusi OB, Ajayi FA, Asunmonu AA, Chukwurimazu O, Ederhion J, et al. Developing frameworks for assessing and mitigating bias in ai systems: A case study on ensuring fairness in AI diagnostic tools through diverse training datasets to prevent misdiagnosis in underrepresented populations. South Asian Research Journal of

Engineering and Technology. 2025;7:33–48

[31] Dutchen S The importance of nuance. Harvard Medicine Magazine [Internet]. 2019. Available from: https://magazine.hms.harvard.edu/articles/importance-nuance [Accessed: 2025-August-13]

[32] Burlina P, Joshi N, Paul W, Pacheco KD, Bressler NM. Addressing artificial intelligence bias in retinal diagnostics. Translational Vision Science & Technology. 2021;**10**(2):13

[33] Stoyanovich J, Howe B, Jagadish HV, Miklau G. Panel: A debate on data and algorithmic ethics. Pvldb. 2018;**11**(12):2165–2167

[34] Raizman E, Peng Y, Deng A. Towards equitable diagnosis: Bias evaluation and mitigation in skin cancer classification. In: Proceedings of the 2024 IEEE Conference on Computational Intelligence in Bioinformatics and Computational Biology (CIBCB); 27-29 August 2024; Natal, Brazil. IEEE; 2024. p. 1–9

[35] European Union. The artificial intelligence act. The EU AI Act Newsletter [Internet] 2021. Available from: https://artificialintelligenceact.eu/ [Accessed: 2025-August-19]

[36] U.S. Food and Drug Administration. Proposed regulatory framework for modifications to artificial intelligence/machine learning-based software as a medical device 2019 [Internet]. 2019. Available from: https://www.fda.gov/files/medical%20devices/published/US-FDA-Artificial-Intelligence-and-Machine-Learning-Discussion-Paper.pdf [Accessed: 2025-August-19]

[37] U.S. Food and Drug Administration. Artificial intelligence/machine learning (AI/ML)-based software as a medical device (SaMD) action plan 2021. [Internet]. 2021. Available from: https://www.fda.gov/medical-devices/software-medical-device-samd/artificial-intelligence-software-medical-device [Accessed: 2025-August 19]

[38] World Health Organization. Ethics and governance of artificial intelligence for health: WHO guidance [Internet]. 2021. Available from: https://iris.who.int/bitstream/handle/10665/341996/9789240029200-eng.pdf [Accessed: 2025-August-20]

[39] World Health Organization. Regulatory considerations on artificial intelligence for health [Internet]. 2023. Available from: https://iris.who.int/bitstream/handle/10665/373421/9789240078871-eng.pdf [Accessed: 2025-August-20]

[40] UNESCO. Recommendations on the Ethics of Artificial Intelligence [Internet]. 2021. Available from: https://unesdoc.unesco.org/ark:/48223/pf0000381137/PDF/381137eng.pdf.multi [Accessed: 2025-August-20]

[41] McCradden MD, Anderson JA, Stephenson AE, Drysdale E, Erdman L, Goldenberg A, et al. A research ethics framework for the clinical translation of healthcare machine learning. The American Journal of Bioethics. 2022;**22**:8–22

[42] Rincón EHH, Jimenez D, Aguilar LAC, Flórez JMP, Tapia ÁER, Peñuela CLJ. Mapping the use of artificial intelligence in medical education: A scoping review. BMC Medical Education. 2025;**25**(1):526

Chapter 4

The Moral and Ethical Implications in the Implementation of Personalized Medicine

Priya Hays

Abstract

This chapter underscores the ethical and moral implications of personalized medicine (PM), which has a certain degree of broad implementation in scientific research, medicine, and healthcare. When the field was in its early stages, bioethical scholars analyzed the challenges of PM and discussed extensively its potential to advance healthcare. However, as described here, the moral and ethical caveats are considered by scholars of PM in the context of philosophical frameworks of Immanuel Kant, the phenomenologists (Merleau-Ponty), and poststructuralism (Michel Foucault), as well as sections on the causal fairness model and the ethics of precision oncology (umbrella and basket trials). The chapter concludes with a discussion on the warnings for preventing structural racism in PM and a systematic review contributing to making the term precise.

Keywords: personalized medicine, bioethics, Kant, phenomenology, causal fairness model, poststructuralism, precision oncology

1. Introduction

Personalized medicine (PM), the tailoring of medications according to the unique genetic and molecular profiles of patients, is, safe to say, implemented in mainstream medicine and scientific research. We are, according to Jeungst et al., "after the Revolution" [1]. Many clinical trials are designed in umbrella and basket forms (TAPUR, NCI-MATCH); targeted therapies and cancer immunotherapies in the PM paradigm are standard of care for oncology patients; liquid biopsy has proven to have analytic and clinical utility; and pharmacogenomics is viewed as a valid way of preventing adverse drug reactions.

However, as bioethicists and scholars have shown, the implementation of PM has come with numerous ethical and social concerns, issues, and problems that warrant active investigation into developing moral and ethical frameworks for addressing these issues [2]. The field is defined as much by its challenges as by its advances. As its proponents first articulated, healthcare today is in a crisis—being reactive, inefficient, and excessively focused on treating late-stage disease—with the answer being a personalized, predictive, preventive, and participatory medicine. Translational genomic medicine, the output of the Human Genome Project, became the strategy for implementing genetic biomarker testing and whole genome sequencing. According to Jeungst et al., each of these attributes – personalized, predictive, preventive, and participatory – comes with its caveats [1]. Prediction brings the risk of medicalization and the stigmatization of the vulnerable through increased clinical surveillance, with the psychosocial costs of labeling people as unhealthy. Prevention may prevent the clinical sequelae of a genetic vulnerability without addressing the underlying causes, and the concept of prevention can encompass forms of social advancement through biomedical manipulation, with the transfer of ethical responsibility for potentially unjust uses of enhancement from researchers to providers. Personalization runs the risk of genetic reduction, whereby consumer genomics reinforces socially ascribed identities and reinscribes labels onto genes. There is also the case of genomic privacy, the risks associated with incidental findings, patient preferences for the "right to know," informed consent, and problematics associated with data sharing and polygenic genomic variants [3]. Data sharing holds the specter of stigmatization as well, since unintended secondary uses of data and breaches in privacy may result from the identification of de-identified data. Privacy concerns arise, leading to the creation of a Data Sharing Privacy Test to facilitate data sharing privacy and require higher protection of an individual's data. Genetic exceptionalism would mandate that the genome is revealing about one's identity and characteristics. The need for genomic privacy must be balanced by the need for large-scale sharing of data. Whole exome sequencing (WES) can strain the physician–patient relationship by shifting more responsibility and expectation onto patients. The return of results also poses ethical concerns in that variants of uncertain significance (VUS) may arise, which have ambiguous interpretations in terms of clinical benefit and whether patients need to know or whether findings are clinically actionable. Issues regarding patient preference and the "right not to know" are central. The return of germ line variants leads to ethical concerns about whether the patient's family needs to know (Hays 2021). McGowan et al. reiterate these concerns in terms of ethical and social issues for PM in oncology and provide an analysis of informed consent for "(1) informed consent, (2) privacy, confidentiality, and disclosure of test results, (3) access to clinical genomic testing and therapies, and (4) the costs of scaling up targeted cancer therapies" [4].

This chapter consists of a literature review of the moral and ethical frameworks guiding the transformation of healthcare and medicine through PM. Philosophers such as Immanuel Kant, Maurice Merleau-Ponty, and Michel Foucault are reflected upon in the context of the personalized and moral issues in the use and application of big data, the formation of the personalized individual, and whether the rational, autonomous Kantian subject is relevant and valid for the new model of personhood as conceived by PM.

Methods: A PubMed, Google, and Google Scholar search with the terms "Moral" and "Ethical" and "Implications" and "Personalized Medicine" or "Philosophical Frameworks" or "Precision Oncology" was conducted, with the exclusion of the terms "Health Economics" and "Literary Criticism."

1.1. Moral and ethical frameworks relevant for PM

The principles of biomedical ethics are autonomy, nonmaleficence, beneficence, and justice, as articulated by Beauchamp and Childress. Recent reports have shown that medical ethics has great relevance for PM. The revealing of an individual's genetic data includes the need for the patients' right to make choices about the risks and benefits of receiving data from their genetic testing. Avoiding harm also means understanding the risks and benefits of receiving targeted therapies and immunotherapies. Beneficence has the strong implication that PM drugs improve outcomes based on individual characteristics, and justice emphasizes fairness and equity in the distribution of resources for all socioeconomic populations and access to genetic testing.

Critical issues such as unnecessary worry, anxiety, and moral burden resulting from genomic testing, as part of ELSI, need to be addressed as well. Difficulty and expense in treatment could lead to the marginalization of patient populations. Psychosocial risks, including distress, anxiety, confusion, as well as stigmatization and discrimination, may have a detrimental effect on the quality of the decision-making process. Employment and insurer discrimination are also risks. Issues of the "right not to know" and the choice not to disclose information arise when family members may need to be informed regarding preventable or treatable diseases. Screening for genetic diseases raises the specter of eugenics. Disclosing the return of results is also a concern since many variants have uncertain significance, especially considering complex disorders such as cancer, with the expectation that potentially clinically significant information can be found. Data integrity must also be preserved since data sharing, portability, analysis, and translation of data are components of the PM paradigm. As Sarwar posits, "[t]he proper translation of genotyping is critical in the era of PM." Additionally, education is needed for participation in large-scale sequencing efforts. EHRs that house patient and clinical data are sources of information for use by clinicians and genomic researchers. Genetic data are unique in that it relates to the person, but also to family members and the community, and respect for privacy emerges as a central concern. HIPAA becomes relevant in the PM workflow, even if genetic data are temporarily anonymized but linked to the patient with the instruction of early identification of increased risk to allow for the necessary steps to reduce risks [5].

Ravan et al. have an elegant articulation of Kant and the novel medicine. For novel medicine, such as PM, "we need an always-renewing and critical framework of ethics." Participatory or P4 medicine can lead to healthism, or health anxiety caused by patient overburden in the individual attending to and being active in their own care. With the expansion of healthcare and its maintenance to families, communities, and society, leading to a sense of biological citizenship – which scholars have termed biopower – the individual is reduced to their healthy or sick body, resulting in the loss of the lived narrative of illness. According to Ravan et al., "health anxiety is opposed to the moral responsibility of medicine to benefit individuals and prevent harm." With unique treatment based on genomic, race, and gender profiles and opportunities leading to patient-centered care, there are problems with resource allocation emanating from PM drugs being expensive and proving to be a financial burden on governments [6]. As the authors state regarding Kant,

> *As Immanuel Kant in Groundwork for Metaphysics of Morals mentioned, acting based on the superior principle of ethics is tied to the freedom of human beings. This means that only the one who is liberated from extrinsic determinants of action acts in compliance with the intrinsic principle of ethics, which is acceptable by all*

> *rational agents. This intrinsic principle is: "act only in accordance with that maxim through which you at the same time can will that it become a universal law [6].*

Abettan and Weili undertake a phenomenological-hermeneutic analysis based on Heideggerian and post-Heideggerian philosophy on the nature of objectivity, subjectivity, the inner world, and the outer world (Being and Time) in the context of PM's impetus for determining the unique nature of individuals. They explain that PM must reverse its concept of personhood and adopt the persona of becoming him or herself (the human being is always distant from itself, never coinciding with itself, and always dwelling near the world instead of being one of the many objects that make up the world) in a temporal fashion. PM becomes "as a part of the dialectic between explanation and understanding," whereby the means and limits of the binary choice between empowerment and burden foster autonomy. Merleau-Ponty expanded on this notion of objectivity–subjectivity with the concept that the "body identifies with the subject," and there is no subjective body in opposition to the objective one. They call for a sociological reflection to occur with an objectiveness of the individual through data for an accurate understanding of personhood. As they state,

"This paradigmatic example reveals that there is no subjective body in opposition to an objective one, but that the body identifies with the subject; or, conversely, that the subject shares the kind of being of the body" [7].

Peebles et al. expound upon the notion they developed of causal fairness as the basis for the socially responsible use of precision medicine. While whole-genome sequencing promises to increase well-being, it also risks "perpetuating psychological essentialism" and "potentially justifying inequality." Causal fairness constitutes a model whereby, in the context of a dearth of relevant strategies to tackle race in genetic medicine, individual-level social processes are deeply embedded in surrounding political, economic, and social structures that further perpetuate and reinforce these biases in individuals. They develop a novel strategy consisting of "(1) a data-driven method for the detection of causal fairness and unfairness in precision health contexts, and (2) an ethical framework for determining when (if ever) it is morally permissible to use a racial classification in population health research." Kidney disease, for example, in African American patients, is associated causally with genetics, but systemic racism could serve as a probabilistic cause as a result of being Black, distinguishing between biological category and social phenomenon. The authors point out the example of the correlation between windshield wipers and the use of an umbrella, which disappears over time when restricted to cases only when it is raining. They also state that "we may not be especially concerned with avoiding the use of genetic predictors of disease whose predictive accuracy is largely due to a socio-causal pathway from the presence of the genetic feature to the protected characteristic and then to the presence of the disease." A genetic feature may lead to patterned racialization, which, in turn, may be responsible for a person's higher likelihood of developing a disease. Strong evidence for this process may redress health inequalities in a salutary way. They also discuss relevant moral frameworks associated with the model of causal fairness, including justice (rights of moral status), benevolence (good will toward others), and trustworthiness (state of moral and technical competence in the entrusted) to promote good medicine in diverse populations. They posit that it is normally permissible to use race when social determinants of health are sufficiently engaged and the medical ends cohere with the aim of medicine: harm minimization. The authors conclude,

> *The causal fairness (CF) model demonstrates that, with sufficient data, researchers can measure whether the inductive use of a particular genomic trait in a clinical context is fair to members of socially salient groups that may be more or less likely to possess that trait. The race-in-medicine (RIM) normative framework proposes that it is morally permissible to use a racial classification in medicine just in case population descriptors do not obscure the role of social factors, best cohere with the aim of the research, and comport with just legal policies that inform medicine [8].*

1.2. Ethics and precision oncology

The recent development and clinical implications of targeted therapies and cancer immunotherapies within the PM paradigm fall into the categories of immune checkpoint inhibitors, bispecific antibodies, antibody–drug conjugates, and chimeric antigen T-cell therapies. These advancements have led to numerous reviews acknowledging the need for proposing and adopting moral and ethical frameworks to mitigate the tangential yet adverse consequences of administering these therapies. The most prominent adverse events include hematologic side effects, cytokine release syndrome, neurotoxicity, and immune-related adverse events affecting organ systems such as the lungs, kidneys, and gastrointestinal tract. Concerns have been raised about mitigating the consequences of these adverse events. In the clinic, additional concerns include issues such as nonresponders, intrinsic and acquired drug resistance, and off-target toxicities associated with these cancer immunotherapies. Liquid biopsy, or circulating tumor DNA analysis, has also emerged within the paradigm of personalized and precision medicine, leading to the development of prognostic and predictive biomarkers such as minimal residual disease and ctDNA levels, which predict overall survival and objective response rates. Next-generation sequencing represents an advancement in the PM paradigm, enabling the discovery of clinically actionable alterations for genetic testing, the prescribing of targeted PM therapies, and the development of biomarkers such as tumor mutational burden. However, concerns surrounding the sensitivity, specificity, and accuracy of PM technologies continue to arise.

McGowan et al. conducted a qualitative study of stakeholders (promoters, monitors, and providers) in PM and elicited the views of these stakeholders through interviews. Their focus was precision oncology, a site where the promise of PM can be realized, and even during the time of publication of this study (2014), genomics, pharmacogenomics, and PM implementation were considered to have great value for cancer. Comments on PM in oncology ranged from considerable enthusiasm to caution to skepticism. Slow adaptation marked other fields in contrast to cancer with a relatively high rate of integration and accommodation. In predicting tumor agnostic therapies, one participant declared:

> *Our whole approach to treating cancer is going to be turned on its head in the next 5 to 10 years, as we will be defining cancer by its molecular signatures as opposed to its histology, and that we're going to be targeting the tumors based on their molecular signatures,*

However, among the participants, ethical concerns remained. Informed consent was particularly problematic since patients may not have knowledge or expertise in cancer genomics and the distinction between somatic and germ line mutations, the risks of germ line and genetic test results, with the BRCA1 allele being provided as an example. Data privacy was also discussed, as patients may be wary that genomic information, when stored in EHRs, runs the risk of employer and insurer access; however, these concerns may be outweighed if cancer treatment outcomes are improved. Access to PM testing may be limited on a population-wide scale, and the high expense and lack of insurance coverage for some targeted therapies may preclude the clinical utility of a genomic test. One participant disclosed that we need to be thinking beyond oncology:

> *A lot of money is often targeted towards cancer for obvious reasons, but you know there are other areas of personalized medicine, other fields which do need some funding: cardiovascular, psychiatry, central nervous system diseases, gastrointestinal diseases, for example. So I don't think it should be particularly targeted towards one particular area, for example cancer. I think it needs to be much broader [3].*

The development and implementation of umbrella and basket trials, two categories of clinical trial designs for precision oncology (PM applications to cancer), were accompanied by concerns over their scientific validity, risk–benefit balance, and informed consent. Together, they form master protocols, whereby multiple tumors in multiple patients harboring distinct molecular profiles can be targeted to determine clinical efficacy for multiple therapies. In a basket trial, with NCI-MATCH being an example, patients with various solid tumors can be enrolled with a targeted therapy according to their alteration. In an umbrella trial, with LUNG-MAP being an example, targeted therapies are matched to a mutation in a tumor, and subsets of tumors grouped together facilitate the evaluation of multiple therapies. As Strzebonska and Waligora highlight, concerns regarding scientific validity and risk–benefit considerations are significant. Scientific validity is a measure of the clinical benefit of a targeted therapy and "one of the essential ethical requirements as the overarching goal of a clinical trial is to provide evidence that can support clinical decision-making." The scientific validity of a basket or umbrella trial is uncertain when considering intratumoral heterogeneity and intertumoral heterogeneity (a tumor and its metastasis), which account for the complexity of a tumor. If not considered, the reliability of the scientific findings may be diminished, and the result may be treatment failure. The reliability of findings may also be undermined by insufficient patient accrual. The risk–benefit ratio of a trial is also central and considers the protection of patients through the bioethical principles of beneficence and nonmaleficence. The authors argue that "the direct benefit achieved by participants of umbrella and basket trials is arguable" since surrogate endpoints are considered over long-term clinical outcomes, but collateral benefit is achieved by the screening of thousands of patients for these protocols. Other risks involved include the patients' coping with incidental findings [9].

1.3. Poststructuralism and recent trends in PM

The relevance of the Kantian framework and traditional biomedical ethics is less certain for personalized and precision medicine; as these genomic technologies evolve, the rational autonomous individual becomes intertwined in contexts defined by stratification and other forms of medicalized grouping.

Personalized medicine, or precision medicine, has entered mainstream scientific research and medical practice in medical centers. Genomic medicine, consisting of genetic testing, whole genome sequencing, and WES, is also part of patient care, and genomic results are being integrated into electronic health records for clinicians.

Many of the problems that may be inherent in the implementation of precision medicine possibly derive from implicit notions of hierarchy embedded in the stratification of adaptive clinical trials, which put some patients at unease—and justifiably so. Targeted therapies, clinically rigorous and sound forms of treatment as shown through studies, are implicitly undermined by the language itself, becoming metaphorical terms for human attack, albeit unwittingly.

The concept of social organization, as embedded in medical activities and scientific research, and the implicit engagement with terminology of attack, was theorized by philosophers in the structuralist and poststructuralist traditions. Medicine and scientific research became the focus of their analysis, and their research revealed nineteenth-century pamphlets on hygiene and maternal and infant care that had very little basis in the scientific method or medical reasoning as it is understood today, but formed the underpinnings of a social structure that inherently enforced conformity and hierarchy.

Precision medicine may have inherited this and reflected this categorization of individuals and the implicit metaphor of attack, as well as genetic testing, and the sequencing of mutations may become another clinical tool that codifies abnormalities among individuals and society. The community of PM scholars and patient advocates may need to come to terms with the theoretical and empirical aspects of the field, as well as the less-than-beneficial social and medical consequences it could cause. While the field has matured, the potential negative consequences should be averted for the individual, the focus of PM's care.

Michel Foucault, one of the most prominent poststructuralists and cultural historians, developed the methods of archeology and genealogy for uncovering the epistemological basis of the hidden structures and systems of thought underlying institutions and social processes, such as the penal system and medical clinic. A notable few of his precepts can help in understanding the moral and ethical implications of patient monitoring (PM). The subject of one of his essays was Jeremy Bentham's panopticon, the prison structure wherein prisoners would be under active surveillance without any knowledge of how or when. Foucault underscored the psychological difficulties and burdens faced by individuals under the circumstances of the panopticon. Patient monitoring is a form of active surveillance in the application of liquid biopsy, as an example, since the temporal heterogeneity of the technology must be captured to determine its predictive and prognostic ability for malignancy and to predict recurrence through minimal residual disease quantification. In this instance, the panopticon must be averted, as the cancer patient must be informed of the surveillance and monitoring potential and its possible adverse implications in adopting the liquid biopsy approach.

In numerous interviews and essays, Foucault expounded on the notion of technologies of self, power, and individual domination. This is particularly thorny when it comes to PM, and one might speculate on the theory that Foucault may have disapproved of PM and wonder whether the PM paradigm would be consistent with the Foucauldian method. However, PM does not concern itself with the prohibition of practices – sexual or otherwise – and this train of thought may have less relevance. PM is participatory medicine, whereby patients and/or consumers take an active role in their health, and the transition from one-size-fits-all leads to proactive or preventive medicine as an advance over reactive medicine, constituting a "care of the self" very much in the Foucauldian sense. The "medical gaze," toward which much of the Foucauldian critique is directed, may also have less relevance since the implementation of PM lies in sequencing and genetic testing.

Vegten has an alternative vision of PM, or precision medicine as he refers to it, and describes the facets of PM as fitting into five medical "cosmologies" as developed by Jewson. The five cosmologies of medicine are Bedside Medicine, Hospital Medicine, Laboratory Medicine, Surveillance Medicine, and E-scaped Medicine, and with each phase comes the effacement of the sick man in medical discourse and practice. Vegten compares Jewson's and others' accounts as intersecting with Foucault's work on the three domains which characterize much of his work: knowledge (The Order of Things), power (Discipline and Punish), and self (Care of the Self). In Precision Medicine, enormous streams of data are required, derived from patient self-monitoring through wearables and smart apps, and transition from genetic testing to genome sequencing to multi-omics. According to Vegten, the result is the reification of the patient as data. Risk and lifestyle become the new cosmology, with new knowledge, new practices of power, and new practices of the self.

> *The emerging Precision Medicine cosmology entails a remapping of illness in large data repositories. Ongoing monitoring and collection of data provides a detailed perspective on illness where inner and outer, body and environment are constantly connected. These new forms of spatialisation and temporalisation gives rise to new knowledge practices.*

Data, rather than being neutral or objective, are never free from the "regulating force of philosophy." Another point made by Vegten is that Foucault, in the 1970s, "showed a growing interest of governments in the health conditions of their populations, leading to the emergence of 'bio-power'. The power of a nations depends on the health of its citizens." Citizens, rather than being seen as individuals or partners, become "digital panopticons," and the role of the individual morphs "as a strategy for making citizens responsible for depositing their data in a digital panopticon, as citizen-managers of their everyday life; empowered to make the 'right' choices." Access to data can be granted to researchers at all strata, as well as citizen-scientists, whose efforts can lead to studies utilizing this information. As Juengst and Prainsack point out, patient empowerment does not automatically become tantamount to positive outcomes, and access to data does not "by definition solve a problem" [10].

> *Individuals are likely to become an exploitable resource, handing off data to external, increasingly powerful parties, while powerful commercial actors are actively involved in the AoU design and in shaping participants' 'lifestyle' choices...a space where practices of freedom are allowed to emerge and where individuals can develop a moral lifestyle, and human individuality may be lost in data streams. Tracking and sharing molecularised self-assessment play an important role in managing our health, thereby created a digital version of a collective Superego.*

Vegten's analysis is certainly relevant, but there are certain problems with it. While he does point out that PM has "lead to a focus on prediction and prevention, providing biomarker-based risk estimates," the focus on the prognostic and predictive ability of PM technologies is more dependent on clinically actionable alterations that are now being implemented through new advances in liquid biopsy and next-generation sequencing, including the relatively wide implementation of WES. Moreover, the emphasis is now on multi-omics strategies that may not reflect any regard for lifestyle or moral outlook and remain within the terrain of the neutral and objective. In fact, despite all of the rhetoric on data reductionism and the inability of patient empowerment and access to data and information to be overall positive, PM has made enormous gains in oncology, pharmacogenomics of cardiovascular medications, as well as genetic testing of heritable diseases such as cystic fibrosis, with new areas emerging such as precision oncology and precision psychiatry. To present any cogent analysis of the caveats of PM through a Foucauldian analysis would have to consider these robust advances in clinical and patient outcomes.

2. Discussion

Despite the eager integration of the PM paradigm in healthcare, controversies still remain, and discussions focus on its moral and ethical implications. As early as 2013, a systematic review was conducted to sharpen the term "personalized medicine" with more precision by analyzing stakeholder discourse, since it remained a vague term in the literature with no distinct definition and was less open to interpretation. They "identified 2,457 articles containing the terms PM in title or abstract. Of those 683 contained a definition of PM and were thus included in [their] review." They derived the ends:

(a) to identify the optimal treatment for each individual patient;

(b) to maximize treatment benefit;

(c) to minimize adverse effects

"as well as the means:

(a) identification of informative biomarkers

(b) stratification of patients."

They concluded that the precising definition is: "PM seeks to improve stratification and timing of health care by utilizing biological information and biomarkers on the level of molecular disease pathways, genetics, proteomics as well as metabolomics," with connotations such as "perfectly tailored" and "patient-centered" being more vague. However, some of their assumptions may be more contestable, since they note that terms such as "research" were not included in the definition because, ostensibly, it did not lead to medical knowledge. The term "drug approval" was also not included as a category relevant to the precise definition of PM [11].

A more recent report articulated on the portent of structural racism in PM. PM may run the risk of perpetuating healthcare inequalities and contributing to a loss of trust in certain minority communities. The connection between structural racism and PM is through the collection of biased health data and their integration into PM initiatives, which "underscore that underappreciation of structural racism by stakeholders involved in the PM ecosystem can be at odds with the ambition of ensuring social and racial justice" [12].

When considering these challenges, concrete and practical recommendations can be offered to potentially resolve the ethical concerns and issues enumerated here (**Table 1**). Jeungst et al. discuss problems such as stigmatization of the vulnerable, increased clinical surveillance, transfer of ethical responsibility to the patient, and reification of social identity through genetic reduction. Additional concerns include the problems of incidental findings, the return of VUS, informed consent, data sharing, data privacy for the protection and deidentification of individual data, and structural racism. Consider the frameworks presented: Kantian ethics, social determinants of health derived from the causal fairness model, the merging of object in the world and subject, and poststructuralist views on the digital panopticon and surveillance in the context of a social structure that mitigates against the hierarchy and conformity of PM technologies. Finally, ensure the scientific validity and low-risk, high-benefit ratio for precision oncology clinical trials, with the application of PM beyond oncology. The steps taken to address these challenges are a function of stakeholder commitment among providers, technology developers, the pharmaceutical industry, and regulators to come to both acknowledgment of these concerns and a consensus on the following: (1) how to regulate the industry to ensure

Philosophical model	Moral and ethical issues of PM	Proposed solution
Kantian	Absolving individual agency through flawed informed consent and clinical trial processes.	Enabling the rational, autonomous individual to make rational decisions regarding their own care.
Phenomenology	The distinction between subject in the world and object distinct.	The technological object has less clear boundaries with the individual and a diminishing lack of connection.
Causal fairness model	Structural racism and relying on genetics as the sole determinant of health.	Applying social determinants of health frameworks to patient care.
Poststructuralism	The intensive reification of the digital, data-driven self; the digital panopticon.	Reduce patients' social anxiety and psychosocial costs by empowering individuals to resist certain social structures.

Table 1.
Key philosophical traditions relevant to PM.

adequate representation of vulnerable populations in clinical trials; (2) how to adequately inform patients of the risks associated with genomic testing for discovering VUS and entering into a precision oncology trial; (3) how to lessen the risk of surveillance of data generated by PM apps, and (4) how to perform liquid biopsies only as necessitated by clinical need rather than solely for research purposes. A Kantian framework would elucidate the rational, autonomous individual, empowering the individual patient to make rational decisions. Social determinants of health, as a function of the causal fairness model, serve as a powerful framework for addressing the specter of structural racism and ensuring fair representation in clinical trials. Phenomenology presents a version of the embodied person that enables the distinction between subject and object to be broken, offering a framework whereby individuals are connected to digital PM technologies. Poststructuralism is powerful for addressing the societal footprint of the moral and ethical implications of PM, wherein the potentially subversive effects of the digital panopticon and technological surveillance are mitigated. This enables PM to free patients from social anxiety, thereby reducing the psychological costs of these innovations.

3. Conclusion

In conclusion, the moral and ethical implications of PM are varied and addressed very extensively in the literature. This review takes into account the views of bioethicists, philosophers, and other commentators to address the actual issues and problems at stake and presents a cogent assessment of their origin and how philosophers in the Kantian, phenomenological, and Foucauldian traditions focus on them and clearly articulate a vision for the problems attendant with PM. With consensus and acknowledgment from the key stakeholders, actionable recommendations are presented with these traditions in mind, as well as novel understandings for approaching them to be implemented responsibly.

Conflict of interest

The author declares no conflict of interest.

Author details

Priya Hays
Geisel School of Medicine at Dartmouth College, Hanover, NH, United States

*Address all correspondence to: priya.hays@outlook.com

References

[1] Juengst ET, Settersten Jr RA, Fishman JR, McGowan ML. After the revolution? Ethical and Social challenges in 'personalized genomic medicine'. Personalized Medicine. 2012;**9**(4): 429–439.

[2] Fierz W. Challenge of personalized health care: To what extent is medicine already individualized and what are the future trends? Medical Science Monitor: International Medical Journal of Experimental and Clinical Research. 2004;**10**:RA111–23.

[3] Hays P. Advancing Healthcare Through Personalized Medicine. Second ed. Cham, Switzerland: Springer Nature; 2021.

[4] McGowan ML, Settersten Jr RA, Juengst ET, Fishman JR. Integrating genomics into clinical oncology: Ethical and social challenges from proponents of personalized medicine. Urologic Oncology: Seminars and Original Investigations. 2014;**32**(2): 187–192.

[5] Sarwar E. Ethical, Social and Public Health implications. Cham, Switzerland: Springer Nature; 2023.

[6] Ravan N, Hasanzad M, Larijani B, and Namazi H. Ethical Concerns in Novel Medicine. In Hasanzhad, M. A Glimpse at Medicine in the Future. Cham, Switzerland: Springer Nature; 2024. pp. 201–212.

[7] Abettan C, Welie JVM. The impact of twenty-first century personalized medicine versus twenty-first century medicine's impact on personalization. Philosophy, Ethics, and Humanities in Medicine. 2020; **15**(1):11.

[8] Peebles IS, Kinney DB, Foster-Hanson E. Systematic decision frameworks for the socially responsible use of precision medicine. NPJ Genomic Medicine. 2024;**9**(1):46.

[9] Strzebonska K, Waligora M. Umbrella and basket trials in oncology: Ethical challenges. BMC Medical Ethics. 2019;**20**(1):58.

[10] Vegter MW. Towards precision medicine; a new biomedical cosmology. Medicine, Health Care and Philosophy. 2018;**21**(4):443–456.

[11] Schledgen S, et al. What is Personalized Medicine. Sharpening A Vague Term in the Literature. BMC Medical Ethics. 2013;**14**:1-12.

[12] Genevieve LD, Martani A, Shaw D, Elger BS, Wangmo T. Structural racism in precision medicine: Leaving no one behind. BMC Medical Ethics. 2020; **21**(1):17.

Chapter 5

Perspective Chapter: Are We All in Clone Club? Bioethical Insights on Genetic Manipulation and Evolution from Pop Culture as a Public Sphere

Yvette Koepke

Abstract

As an extreme horizon, human cloning offers a locus to analyze the ethics of all forms of genetic manipulation writ large. Gauging and engaging the public in deliberation around such momentous and controversial technologies has been widely advocated. This chapter will examine the implications of popular representations, which both reflect and shape cultural attitudes and meanings of not just cloning, but also genes, biomedical science, evolution, and bioethical decision-making itself. Texts create a shared space to explore and even experience what-if scenarios in their full complexity and emotional resonance. This public sphere does the work of critique as well as theorizing by imagining (im)possibilities. Specifically, representations of human clones and cloning show how we are all subject to the circulation of data, technologies, and capital that can reinforce systems of historical oppression, yet move beyond such critique to intervene in bioethical debate and envision potential models of action and alliance that do not rely on an individual "natural" identity or simply reject technological science.

Keywords: cloning, postmodern identity, popular culture, public policy, bioethics, genetics, evolution, global capitalism, narrative, technology

1. Introduction

As a moral and technological horizon, human reproductive cloning is arguably the ultimate test case for applied bioethics. The United States Congress Human Cloning Prohibition Act of 2003 asserts, "Few issues have ever created such a unified public opposition as the possibility of producing human beings who are genetically identical to an already existing individual." It is arguably the clearest instance of the "Frankenstein syndrome," in which "the myth is either accepted as literal truth or categorically rejected as nonsense" [1], thereby foreclosing meaningful exploration of the complexities ignored by either stance. Analyzing the popular culture meanings attached to cloning avoids this oversimplification, with implications for public attitudes and decision-making, as well as broader underlying understandings of genetics and evolution. Representations of clones, such as the popular TV series *Orphan Black,* reflect and shape cultural attitudes toward controversial techniques, but also express the inauthenticity and fragmentation of global postmodern society, as well as the widespread "geneticization" of all identities. Representations of clones and cloning provide a public space for shared critical, ethical examination of the ways that the circulation of data, technologies, and capital can reinforce systems of historical oppression. Such representations further offer crucial insights in moving beyond such critique to intervene in common bioethical debates and theorize potential models of action and alliance that do not rely on an individual, stable "natural" identity or simply reject technological science.

2. Complicating meanings of clones

Over its four seasons, the television series *Orphan Black* (2013–2017) garnered rave critical reviews and soaring ratings, with a spin-off, *Orphan Black: Echoes*, in 2023. The titular character, Sarah Manning, whose name positions her as an Every-Man, learns that she is part of a group of diverse clones who begin to work together to uncover the truth of their creation and protect themselves against groups that want to eliminate or use them. This representation reflects, as well as shapes, changing views of cloning and its broader underlying logic of genetic manipulation, including research such as therapeutic cloning, screening, engineering, and editing. For example, it refutes the genetic determinism dictating the admonitory dystopia of *Gattaca* (1997), divided into "in-valids" and "valids," and humorously depicted as an infinite number of exact "copies" needed for a hard-pressed "family man" to "get more out of life" in *Multiplicity* (1996). Sarah states, "They're not me. They're completely different people." Fundamentally, the series elicits viewer recognition of the full and unique humanity of each clone, intervening in common bioethical arguments not only about cloning itself but also about bioethics and where ethical decision-making occurs.

Every clone is radically unique in style, personality, sexuality, and status: cop to con artist, lesbian glasses-wearing intellectual to stay-at-home soccer mom. Not simply life choices, this profound variance in capacities insists upon the individual identity of each clone. This uniqueness helps communicate scientific facts often glossed over: differences in innumerable factors building over time – oocyte cytoplasm, epigenetics, environment, upbringing, experiences, neuroplasticity, to name several – overlay DNA sameness, such that clones would be less alike than the "natural" clones of identical twins [2, 3]. *Orphan Black* therefore denies the hierarchical logic of *Multiplicity*'s husband-clones, signaled in the movie poster by #1's (sexual) possession of his wife as well as by the lower position of the second part of the word and the inverted "i" representing the secondary (lesser) carbon copies. This is the same logic invoked in calls to prohibit cloning because of its threat to the natural family order instantiated by sexual reproduction, as articulated in the National Bioethics Advisory Commission's 1997 report [4]. Further, the show raises questions about the universality of deep-seated emotional responses like "repugnance" and their use as metonyms of ethical meaning or judgment.

Focus on the clones themselves as the hero breaks from prior cautionary representations that mirrored profound societal unease. The show pointedly rebuts staple features of these representations, such as lack of emotion or sameness, which inform colloquial usage of the word "clone" and nightmare scenarios like an army of Hitlers that reiterated rigid gender norms at the same time that they signaled the essential wrongness of cloning itself. Indeed, the relative lack of response to recent reported breakthroughs in human cloning, such as the 2013 production of stem cells from cloned human embryos by a team at Oregon Health & Science University, suggests that the oft-invoked universality of condemnation may be unhelpfully reductive. Shifting attitudes may have been shaped by a reconceptualization of cloning as a technology: a form of biomedical research rather than a horrifying mode of reproduction, and "it is possible that the decades of frightening stories have counterintuitively had the effect of making the public more accepting of, or even indifferent to, real-life developments."[4] Nor does *Orphan Black* locate cloning elsewhere, in a different or *Future Shock* dystopic time or space, but in "Generica." Cloning becomes a fait accompli driven by high-tech profit, its illegality beside the point and of no help whatever to the clones themselves. The show thereby crystallizes the myriad challenges and limitations of prohibition and regulation, including how bans encourage privatized funding and thereby may have the opposite effect intended by hamstringing the role of the public sphere, as seen in the history of reproductive medicine more broadly [5].

Orphan Black critically examines the authoritative roles commonly given to genetics, medicine, and science. This authoritative gaze has historically been particularly oppressive to women, as suggested by Wesley Anderegg's sculpture, "The First Human Clone" (2010). A "primitive" figure sits in a traditional circus wagon displayed behind metal bars, its monstrosity apparent in green skin, a wide mouth with too many teeth, and extranumerary deformed toes and fingers, as well as a lack of physical or social gender markers other than breasts. Cloning creates "freaks," whether by failure to control phenotype, as in the sculpture, or by the covert monitoring and testing, which are simply extensions of the cloning procedure itself. Alison's deepest fear is that her children will discover that she is a "freak." The impact of negative societal attitudes (the gaze at the freak show) as a potential harm to clones is sometimes brought into ethical debate in terms of prejudice and discrimination, while the potential harm of internalization and self-perception is commonly overlooked but foregrounded in, for example, Mary Shelley's *Frankenstein* (1818). Ostensibly the most "normal" of the clones, Alison is also the most seemingly paranoid and repeatedly claims that they are "lab rats" in someone's "experiment." Alison expresses what has been termed "the principle of dangerous science": a technological inevitability driven by potential intellectual or economic value, which overrides potential concerns about harm or ethics [6]. The fact that the unsophisticated suburban soccer mom is proved correct illustrates the societal normalization of profound technoscientific intervention. Indeed, clones highlight the widespread "geneticization" of all identities in an era of forensic DNA analysis, popular genealogy testing, mass genetic screening, the Human Genome Project, and growing use of reproductive technologies.

The series revisits familiar concerns about profit- and power-hungry bioscientific corporations like the shiny, fictional Dyad Institute. Equally, though, it rejects the refuge of untouched, sanctified nature (and "natural" sexual reproduction), the position of the fundamentalist religious group known as the Proletheans. Though diametrically opposed, Dyad and the Proletheans equally "play God," one of the most common condemnations of not just reproductive but also therapeutic cloning and gene editing like CRISPR [7]. From the Prolethean perspective, which posits an original ideal predicated on willful (Lethe-an) forgetfulness or denial of scientific advances, a clone "impostor" – referred to as "it" and "fingernail clippings" – is "nothing," not "real." Thus, the Proletheans have trained another clone, Helena, to assassinate the rest of the "dirty copies." Helena is an avenging angel, inscribed in the wing self-scarification on her back and her halo of blond curly hair. Emerging from the dim, curved womb of a ship's hold after ritualized purification-cum-healing, Helena embodies the etymological and mythic meaning of her name: she is the "light." Helena contrasts with Sarah on both counts: she is not an orphan, with a quasi-religious father-figure and the "family" of Proletheans, nor is she "black" in feature (Helena's skin and hair are very pale, and she wears white) or supposed moral standing.

The danger of this logic is graphically manifested in the visceral brutality of Helena's killings, but also in the damage to Helena herself. She is a hunter who is hunted, a haunter of the shadows who cannot be "made" into an angel without being an animal who devours food and is physically caged like a lab rat by her so-called "father," who proclaims, "If you protect this forgery [another clone], you're no better than they are." Helena being dragged to her cage echoes Sarah being drugged and taken from her bed for medical testing. Helena calls Sarah to free her from the cage, just as Sarah had earlier called on Helena to "save" her from Dyad capture. Helena is able to stand in for Sarah precisely because of Dyad's violence, in the form of the black bag over her head rendering them interchangeable. The narrative momentum of the entire first season culminates in discovering the "lie" obscured by the trappings of "informed consent" in the contracts offered to each clone. "Pure" science is no more of a solution than "pure" nature. But neither is "no" science the answer: significantly, another clone – Cosima, a genetics grad student researcher – uses science to work from "inside," and Sarah worries about "scientists more than science." In short, the show insists that medical scientists acknowledge situated interestedness in order to act ethically, thereby offering a more relevant vision for an increasingly technoscientific future [8].

3. Critiquing geneticization and gender

Moreover, it is the prevailing geneticized model of identity, not just hyperbolic villains like Dyad, that reduces people to barcodes, to readily circulatable data. DNA is a fetish, a cultural icon that has "come to stand for something's essence" and secures molecular biomedicine as "the dominant science of the second half of the twentieth century" [9]. Whether this information is put to good or ill use or "owned" by Dyad or by the "sovereign" subject herself, it instantiates a prior separation between self and body. In this way, we are all clones. Anderegg's sculpture was part of the Yellowstone Art Museum's 2014 exhibit of portraits, Face to Face. The show's symbolic layers extend its social critique by manifesting anxieties to which we are all subject. The clone orphans express our sense of alienation – fueled by material mobility and the rise of the "virtual," digital world – and our accompanying suspicion that we are interchangeable or expendable. Worse, that we may have been engineered this way to create the *Brave New World* envisioned by Aldous Huxley in 1932. From identity theft to government surveillance, modern society shares with *Orphan Black* an omnipresent and justifiable fear of hidden control. The horror of the literal bar code discovered in the clones' DNA is magnified by the realization that their manipulation, their commodification, really feels like more of the same in the age of "bioinformatics": "Life is information, and this information itself is manipulable, spliceable, rewriteable, translatable, and, in the end, commodifiable" [10]. More concretely, can intentions or goals behind cloning be identified that would be fundamentally different from any of those found in natural reproduction? [11] And can we predict the responses of future generations either to genetic interventions or forbearance from screening, manipulations, and so on? [10] More subtly, the exaggerated stereotypes embodied by various clones demonstrate the profound pressure to fit certain roles, but at the same time reveal the performative construction of those roles and the potential to rescript them. In this way, the series stresses the autonomy and "open future" whose attributed compromise has been central to some ethical condemnations of reproductive cloning [12, 13]. Even Helena, whose very existence has been brutally reduced to an object or means in Kantian terms, remains a unique subject and human actor.

If *Multiplicity* expressed societal anxieties about how to "be a man" when that role expanded beyond the workplace, *Orphan Black* expresses societal anxieties about how to "be a woman." The narrative intercuts the caging of Helena and the police closing in on Sarah with Alison's ambush by a circle of her priest, husband, and friends. Alison replies: "I thank you. For scrutinizing every detail of my life, since I moved into this fish bowl. You have pried and snooped and gossiped about me, like I was your own personal laboratory subject. How would you like it if I turned your life inside out?" The genetic intervention that has made her life a "freak show" to be "monitored" is reciprocal with this mundane "intervention." Both share the same justification by other's judgments about her best interest. The paternalism of both is highlighted by their gendering and calls attention to possible paternalism in arguments projecting the exploitation of women specifically in cloning processes. Far from docile conformity *à la* Huxley, Alison is at the center of what they call "Clone Club" in an ironic reference to the movie *Fight Club* (1999). This subterranean group of unlikely women meets in the finished basement – the "family room" – of her suburban home. Like the Narrator of *Fight Club*, disaffection drives Alison to violently attack repressive elements, while Sarah can be read as the film's Tyler Durden, her "dark" alter ego. However, Alison does not become Sarah but redeploys and literalizes her own Alison-ness. She tells nosy neighbors that her husband is "tied up" while she's secured him to a chair in her craft room with patterned duct tape; she tells him to think about what he "really want[s] to get off [his] chest" while she drips hot glue from her crafting glue-gun onto it.

Fight Club is a hypermasculine fantasy (tagline: "MISCHIEF. MAYHEM.") of the alienation of the unnamed corporate drone (portrayed by a sallow Edward Norton in shirt and tie) from his fundamental manliness (a grinning, cocky, squared-off Brad Pitt). The background of Norton's "mug shot" in the movie's poster shows him as a wild animal taken from its habitat to live in a globally generic zoo. This fantasy posits an "outside" to the vitiated "support group" self and society. In contrast, Clone Club is queer, with no outside to run to. It's impossible to follow rules you don't know, so Sarah brought her gay foster brother, Felix, to Alison's, causing ongoing reciprocal contamination. As highly stereotyped roles get repeated, they also get repurposed and revisioned. Felix's disguise as Alison's gay "acting coach" turns into Felix doing a "reverse Pygmalion" for her to impersonate Sarah. To go back to her house after she attacked her husband, Alison needs to "fetch [him] something gay" to reprise his role, while Felix instructs Alison to "be a woman": "this is Backstabbing

101." His advice then circulates as a literal inspirational poster that highlights the feminine springtime colors and self-growth motif captured by the tulip print on the wall. Self-growth, tongue-in-cheek, nods to literal self-growth possible through cloning, which may have real consequences for a queer challenge to the latent heterosexism embedded in appeals to natural sexual reproduction [14, 15].

Orphan Black challenges the *Fight Club* split between the two day-and-night sides of the insomniac Narrator. The film builds to the revelation that Durden is "really" the Narrator. Yet none of the sought-after "answers" in *Orphan Black* settle anything; it is instead a series of "middles." Sarah constantly plays catch-up, just like viewers. It's not that she doesn't figure anything out – after all, she learns she's a clone in Episode 2 – but instead that answers become questions: "Every time I think I know something I'm wrong." The narrative only moves forward; the pace accelerates, and the number of narrative strands multiply and ramify with dizzying cuts between locations, last-minute phone calls, and unforeseen events. The first season ends as it began. Again, the impossible enlarges the possible: Sarah sees "herself" turn around and do something unthinkably self-destructive – offer the Dyad contract. At this point, the "informed" viewer asks the same questions as Sarah, extending the slippage between self and "other": Who is this person? Why did she do it? What should I do? This positioning of the viewer communicates the stakes, the uncertainty, and the insufficiency of the concept of "informed consent" in a viscerally affecting way.

4. Rethinking determinism: Implications for bioethics

Knowing that the woman is obviously a clone does not answer these questions. *Orphan Black* offers a contemporary theorization of identity beyond the naturalized "family tree" promised by services like AncestryDNA. However, the information carefully laid out in the Dyad document, even the sequenced genome given to Cosima, does not tell any of them what they should do. The story – which is never only singular – doesn't just need to be told backward, but also forward, by, for, and with each-who-is-also-all of them [16]. The ultimate technology of deliberately designing a human being once again illustrates the "special problem of technology" and its phantasmic lure: wonder, immediacy, certainty, power, distance, self-perpetuation [17]. Each clone is forced to interpret, to act emergently without knowing, to enact lived subjectivity – an elaboration of a feminist ethics focused on the "need to develop a moral analysis that fits the actual world in which we live" [18] rather than abstracted universal principles. This is an ethics that grows out of collective disagreement and deliberation in the public sphere, embodied by the family room and pink burner "clone phones." When Cosima tells Sarah, "We're your biological imperative now," the deterministic phrase produces a horizontally shifting coalition rather than an independent individual or vertically hierarchical reproduction as passing-on-genes. Whereas cloning's disruption of traditional social structures and family roles has featured heavily in ethical critiques, the series explores how becoming an "orphan," removed from the natural family through cloning, may open up alternative modes of filiation – and further, how these could offer feminist resistance to institutionalized patriarchal oppression.

At issue is survival, Sarah's most basic identity, according to her foster mother: "I just wanna know who I am." "You're still you. Remember that. You're a survivor."

Sarah engages in flexible, self-reflexive practice based on her experiential knowledge. The very skills of impersonation and improvisation, developed through the endless struggle – to use a favorite phrase of Darwin – of being "orphan black" or living outside the system, make her "fittest" to respond to the collective "need" by playing other clones to get information, playing the "game" but "changing [it] for everyone" by playing everyone against each other. Streetwise Sarah has lived her life in the shadows, on her own, looking out for herself. Latecomer that she is, Sarah is her namesake, the ironic Biblical matriarch. The conviction that she "came out of the woodwork" like a hidden pest and is not "special" – in other words, the fluid inauthenticity of her self, her acceptance of contingent uncertainty – offers repertoires. Her answer to "What am I gonna do" is, "I don't know how I'm going to play this." Sarah challenges the Prolethian ideology of purity and authenticity, which depends on an origin(al) to devalue and destroy the "impostor." In Clone Club, there are only impostors. Set against the originary "word is light," Sarah is clearly a "forgery," but she is also the forger: the intentions and plans of her creators do not remove her autonomy or decide in advance what is possible, even while they set conditions. Putting this in terms of bioethical debate over cloning: knowledge of the origin(al) may circumscribe a clone's life and place a burden or shadow, but it may equally be inspiring, encouraging, or empowering, and this in itself remains open [19].

Orphan Black likewise critiques the determinism and control of Dyad's "Neolution," or "the new science of self-directed evolution," which overlaps with popular understandings of evolution as well as theorizations of it, like sociobiology. Cosima's invitation to a lecture on "Neolution – Now!" is framed using the authority of her own father-figure: "as a Darwinist [. . .] it would interest you." The Dyad lecturer, Dr. Aldous Leekie, plans to reveal Cosima's "origin" because he believes it will dictate her identity and, therefore, her behavior, such that she will be recruited to Dyad successfully. As an engineered clone, Cosima is but an exaggeration of the underlying logic selling DNA tests or positioning the object of knowledge as a thing instead of an actor [20]. However, the series questions such a reductive facticity. Its overall structure reworks the "origin" through allusive, disordered citation as parts of different stories get uncovered, shared, jumbled, and listened to. This narrative structure further calls attention to "how a story is used on different occasions of its telling" [21], which inflects bioethical analysis. Crucially, it also emphasizes elements of Darwinian evolution that have been replaced by the doctrine of genetics as a master code leading to naturalized good and unquestioned progress [22], namely, variability produced through the effects of environment and development. The ironic play on Dr. Louis Leakey, the famous Darwinian paleoanthropologist who argued for studying primates in their natural habitats, foregrounds this aspect of evolution.

Each episode's title refers to Darwin's *On the Origin of Species* (1859), moving from universally recognized concepts to those less familiar, which insist upon variability and the impact of specific contexts and conditions:

1. Natural Selection

2. Instinct

3. Variation under nature

4. Effects of external conditions
5. Conditions of existence
6. Variations under domestication
7. Parts developed in an unusual manner
8. Entangled bank
9. Unconscious selection
10. Endless forms most beautiful

Darwin repeatedly describes "(en)tangled bank(s)" to counter the notion of "chance" in favor of the "Complex Relations of All Animals and Plants to Each Other in the Struggle for Existence": "It is interesting to contemplate a tangled bank, clothed with many plants of many kinds, with birds singing on the bushes, with various insects flitting about, and with worms crawling through the damp earth, and to reflect that these elaborately constructed forms, so different from each other, and dependent upon each other in so complex a manner, have all been produced by laws acting around us." Yet this same description of an entangled bank, instead of a (grafted) branch, equally refuses the (self-)determinism often ascribed to genes and natural selection and encoded by the etymology of the word "clone," carrying the historical weight of man's mastery over passive vegetative nature. Dyad promulgates this very determinism, implied by its reductive name, which shades into control and absolute, predictable knowledge. Rather, Darwin stresses concrete becoming, multiplicity, and interrelation along surfaces more than causal depth [21, 23]. The textual features reinforce the meaning: the length and complexity of the sentence with its numerous linked dependent clauses; the profuse alliteration, parallelism, and repetition creating connections; the unpredictable activity of the fauna. The emphasis on the esthetic and sensory, and the explicit positioning of the observer's perceptions, reiterates multiplicity of perspectives and layers of meaning, as does the figurative use of "clothed," with its implied agency as well as beauty.

5. Conclusion

Precisely by creating an experiment in which the origin of a new "species" has been rigorously designed and controlled, the series questions the authority of certain knowledge in medicine and ethics. The most carefully controlled and funded scientific research cannot predict the sicknesses suffered by some (not all) of the clones – a key point in calls to prohibit and regulate cloning. "Black sheep," "wild child" Sarah is also "wild type," who has a miraculous daughter against her explicit genetic design. Sarah's birth mother is incredibly revealed to be a Black immigrant who multiply displaces the "origin(al)": a mother who is not-like-her, neither the genetic source nor the intended parent "dreamed about," a splitting in the darkness of her womb beyond the intention and control of the medical scientists, which produces Sarah and Helena. Thus, the singular title of "Orphan Black" refers to both Sarah and Helena. In the opening credits, they are the two "I"s or bars of the "H" that sits at the center of O–R–P–H–A–N, connected and made meaningful only by the double helix serving as the letter's cross-bar, just as all of the individual clones become a distributed cyborg assemblage linked by the "secondary" pink clone phones used to contact one another secretly or in the "black." The sliding music using glissando and the shifting, not-quite-mirror images of the title sequence emphasize movement, processes of multiplying and becoming. Sarah is not split or replaced, like the Narrator in *Fight Club*, but is reflected and refracted.

Rather than the empty sameness of the transparent glass vessels in the title sequence, which are suggestive of laboratory manipulations, Sarah and Cosima see themselves externalized in a mirror as they meet to talk at an everyday bar, and, in turn, see themselves seeing each other as same-and-different. Morality is for "amateurs," "something we all do together," "as a continual interpersonal task of becoming and remaining mutually intelligible." [16] Seeing themselves in and as one another while recognizing that person as "real" – distinct from but sitting next to you – is a complex ethical process, an articulation of embodied, partial, situated knowledge: a view from somewhere to counter objective rationality or the view from above/nowhere [20]. The "self" cannot simply be rooted, nor can it be distinguished from the "other" definitively. If debates and official statements regarding cloning have revealed the seeming impossibility of defining "human dignity" [24, 25], *Orphan Black* points our attention away from individualized uniqueness as the stable ground of identity and toward interrelation as the core of humanity. *Orphan Black* elaborates an "I" and "us" relationship more than an "I" and "you." Sarah asks, "What are we to each other?" and "How many of us are there?" She is implicated quite literally by her fingerprints, her face, her DNA, but finds herself enfolded in a shifting, distributed collective, an "entangled bank," to use Darwin's image, instead of the simplistic stick figures or paper "fortune teller" offered by Helena. Genetic identity is one of the "conditions of existence" but is not determinant. Affiliations are provisional and enacted, neither "freely chosen" without reference to lived conditions nor simply given or predetermined. They are not sisters but "sestra," in Helena's dialect. Material fact falls short of feeling, which is necessarily embodied and ethical [26]: Helena feeling connected to Sarah, Sarah feeling that something is being held back, Alison feeling like it's her own daughter (not Sarah's) who is in danger. Whereas cloning has long signified tyrannical or robotic sameness in popular culture and bioethics, *Orphan Black* imagines how cloning – a specific procedure but also the shared condition of all postmodern, technologically elaborated subjects – can also be "kinda cool," in Cosima's words, by opening up possibilities for the "endless forms most beautiful" of an entangled bank.

Author details

Yvette Koepke
University of North Dakota, Grand Forks, ND, United States of America

*Address all correspondence to: yvette.koepke@und.edu

References

[1] Rollin B. The Frankenstein Syndrome. Cambridge: Cambridge University Press; 1995. p. 241

[2] Pulman B. The issues involved in cloning: Sociology and bioethics. Revue Française de Sociologie. 2007;**48**:129–156. DOI: 10.3917/rfs.485.0129

[3] Johnson G. Soul searching. In M. c. N, Sunstein C, editors Clones and Clones: Facts and Fantasies about Human Cloning. New York: Norton; 1999. p. 67–70

[4] The Witherspoon Council. Special report: The threat of human cloning: Ethics, recent developments, and the case for action. The New Atlantis. 2015;**46**:9–146

[5] Hall SH. Eve redux: The public confusion over cloning. The Hastings Center Report. 2003; **33**(3):11–15. DOI: 10.2307/3528432

[6] Rozell DJ. Dangerous Science: Science Policy and Risk Analysis for Scientists and Engineers. London: Ubiquity Press; 2020. p. 166

[7] Rollin BE. Keeping up with the Cloneses: Issues in human cloning. The Journal of Ethics. 1999; **3**(1):51–71. DOI: 10.1023/A:1009775715165

[8] Brody H. Who gets to tell the story? Narrative in postmodern bioethics. In Lindemann Nelson H, editor Stories and Their Limits. New York: Routledge; 1997. p. 18–30

[9] Comfort N. The Science of Human Perfection: How Genes Became the Heart of American Medicine. New Haven: Yale University Press; 2014. p. 316

[10] Mendieta E. The Philosophical Animal: On Zoopoetics and Interspecies Cosmopolitanism. Albany: State University of New York Press; 2024. p. 266

[11] Davis DS. What's wrong with cloning? Jurimetrics. 1997;**38**(1):83–89

[12] Brock DW. Cloning human beings: An assessment of the ethical issues pro and con. In C NMCS, editor Clones and Clones: Facts and Fantasies about Human Cloning. New York: Norton; 1999. p. 141–164

[13] Glannon W. The ethics of human cloning. Public Affairs Quarterly. 1998; **12**(3):207–305. DOI: 10.1016/s1472-6483(10)62205-5

[14] W.n. Jr E, Stein E, Queer clones. In C NMCS, editor Clones and Clones: Facts and Fantasies about Human Cloning. New York: Norton; 1999. p. 95–113

[15] Tribe L. On not banning cloning for the wrong reasons. In C NMCS, editor Clones and Clones: Facts and Fantasies about Human Cloning. New York: Norton; 1999. p. 221–232

[16] Lindemann Nelson H, Context: Backward, sideways, and forward. In M CRM, editor Stories Matter: The Role of Narrative in Medical Ethics. New York: Routledge; 2002. p. 39–47

[17] Cassell ED. The Nature of Primary Care Medicine. Oxford: Oxford University Press; 1997. p. 206

[18] Sherwin S. No Longer Patient: Feminist Ethics and Health Care. Philadelphia: Temple University Press; 1992. p. 286

[19] Epstein RA. A rush to caution: Cloning human beings. In C NMCS, editor Clones and Clones: Facts and Fantasies about Human Cloning. New York: Norton; 1999. p. 262–279

[20] Haraway D. Situated knowledges: The science question in feminism and the privilege of partial perspectives. In Harding S, editor The Feminist Standpoint Theory Reader. New York: Routledge; 2004. p. 81–102

[21] Frank A. The Wounded Storyteller. Chicago: The University of Chicago Press; 1995. p. 213

[22] Harris J. Enhancing Evolution: The Ethical Case for Making Better People. Princeton: Princeton University Press; 2010. Vol. **242**, p. 2007

[23] Novas C, Rose N. Genetic risk and the birth of the somatic individual. Economy and Society. 2010; **29**(4): 485–513. DOI: 10.1080/0308514005 0174750

[24] Arsanjani MH. Negotiating the UN Declaration on Human Cloning. The American Journal of International Law. 2006; **100**(1):164–179. DOI: 10.2307/ 3518835

[25] Childress JF. Human cloning and human dignity: The report of the President's Council on Bioethics. The Hastings Center Report. 2003; **33**(3): 15–18. DOI: 10.2307/3528433

[26] Morris D. Illness and Culture in the Postmodern Age. Berkeley: University of California Press; 2000. p. 345

Chapter 6

Ethical Hazards of Large Language Models in Primary Care: A Clinician-Focused Update

Michelle Lu, Justin J. Gillette and Thomas F. Heston

Abstract

Large Language Models (LLMs) are transforming clinical workflows in primary care through capabilities like diagnostic support, clinical documentation, and simulated empathetic engagement. Yet, these advancements bring underappreciated ethical hazards that directly impact front-line physicians. Unlike general discussions of AI ethics, this chapter focuses on dilemmas arising with the use of LLMs in real-world primary care: questions of liability when LLM suggestions influence clinical decisions; risks to confidentiality when LLMs interact with protected health information; cognitive offloading that may erode diagnostic skills; disruptions in patient trust when LLMs simulate empathy; and the growing reality of patients turning to generative models as informal therapists. As LLMs are embedded into electronic medical records and clinical apps, physicians must become active ethical agents in how these tools are used. These challenges arise in contexts where regulatory frameworks lag behind technological deployment, placing responsibility squarely on individual clinicians to navigate uncertain ethical terrain. Drawing on current literature and real-world clinical challenges, this chapter proposes a clinician-focused ethical framework to guide the responsible use of LLMs in primary care. This framework addresses both immediate practical concerns—such as informed consent for LLM-assisted care and appropriate documentation of AI involvement—and longer-term questions about professional identity and diagnostic autonomy in an AI-augmented practice environment. The goal is not to demonize these powerful tools but to equip physicians with the necessary conceptual tools, awareness, and decision-making strategies for safe and ethical integration. Ultimately, the foundation of primary care—human judgment, presence, and trust—must remain at the center of clinical decision-making, even in an era augmented by LLMs.

Keywords: Artificial Intelligence, large language models, primary care ethics, clinical decision-making, Generative AI, confidentiality, empathy

1. Introduction

Large language models (LLMs), such as ChatGPT, represent a recent paradigm shift in clinical informatics, with immediate and far-reaching implications for the practice of primary care. These generative models operate by leveraging transformer-based neural network architectures, trained on extensive medical and general-domain corpora, enabling outputs that resemble human reasoning and dialog [1]. In the primary care setting, characterized by longitudinal relationships, diagnostic ambiguity, and high cognitive load, LLMs are already being embedded in tools for documentation automation, differential diagnosis support, prior authorization, and patient communication interfaces.

Despite these utilities, the ethical hazards introduced by LLM deployment are underappreciated by clinicians and underrepresented in guidelines. Unlike algorithmic tools that are rule-based or supervised, LLMs operate in stochastic and opaque ways, with outputs influenced by training biases, prompt phrasing, and model-specific heuristics. In this sense, they blur traditional ethical boundaries: authorship becomes ambiguous, accountability is diffused, and the illusion of understanding may obscure diagnostic uncertainty [2, 3].

Furthermore, their integration into real-time clinical workflows introduces tensions specific to primary care. These include liability ambiguity when clinical actions are influenced by LLM-generated text, erosion of patient trust when empathy is simulated, confidentiality risks arising from model-data interaction, and the potential atrophy of clinical reasoning due to cognitive offloading. For example, recent studies indicate that patients are already using generative models as informal therapists, prompting complex medico-ethical considerations about the scope of practice, consent, and monitoring [4, 5].

This chapter examines these ethical fault lines from the standpoint of the practicing primary care physician. It does not offer a general LLM ethics theory, nor does it advocate for or against the use of LLMs per se. Instead, it identifies five concrete domains where dilemmas arise at the interface of LLMs and clinical reasoning: liability and clinical judgment, confidentiality and trust, erosion of clinical thinking, the physician-patient relationship, and patients' use of LLMs as informal therapists. For each domain, we provide a pragmatic ethical framework for physicians confronted with LLM-integrated tools. The aim is to reinforce the clinician's role as a moral agent, not merely a user, who must evaluate, interpret, and sometimes resist technological interventions. As LLMs become fixtures of the clinical landscape, the ethical center of gravity must remain rooted in human judgment, professional accountability, and the physician-patient relationship.

2. Liability and clinical judgment

"If I Follow the LLM and Get Sued, Who Pays?"

The use of LLMs in clinical reasoning presents a profound ethical and legal inflection point for primary care. At the heart of this transformation arises a novel ethical dilemma: the diffusion of accountability. Historically, medical liability has been grounded in a clinician's autonomous judgment, informed by best practices, clinical training, and professional discretion. However, when a physician acts based on LLM-generated suggestions – particularly from a generative model that offers probabilistic rather than deterministic guidance – the lines of responsibility become blurred [6]. LLMs do not possess agency, yet their outputs may materially influence decision-making in diagnosis, prescribing, and triage. This further demonstrates the profound influence of LLMs in primary care, but one whose accountability remains unassigned.

Unlike traditional clinical decision support systems, which follow transparent if-then logic, LLMs produce outputs based on statistical associations derived from opaque training data [7]. Thus, even when an LLM generates a plausible diagnostic or therapeutic recommendation, its underlying rationale cannot be reliably interrogated or reproduced in clinical practice [8]. Consequently, physicians remain fully liable for medical harm – even when decisions are materially shaped by algorithmic suggestions whose basis cannot be interrogated. This leads to liability asymmetry: the model may substantially inform a clinical decision, yet the legal burden of error and ethical accountability remains exclusively on the clinician. Furthermore, commercial LLM providers often explicitly disclaim medical responsibility in their terms of service, reinforcing that physicians bear full legal exposure – even when model outputs are directly integrated into electronic health record (EHR) interfaces or clinical workflows [9–11]. While regulatory bodies and professional organizations are beginning to develop LLM-specific guidance for healthcare settings, these frameworks remain nascent and have not yet resolved the fundamental question of liability distribution when LLMs materially influence clinical decisions.

Compounding this legal uncertainty is implicit delegation. LLMs generate highly fluent and confident-sounding text, masking significant errors, biases, or omissions rooted in training data skew [11]. In such settings, clinicians may unconsciously defer to LLM suggestions, even if they conflict with their clinical judgment and intuition [9, 12].

This dynamic is particularly hazardous in high-stakes scenarios such as chest pain triage, antibiotic stewardship, or prescribing in polypharmacy contexts. A physician who defers to an LLM-generated differential diagnosis may do so without recognizing the hidden assumptions embedded in the model's output. This risk is heightened under time constraints and cognitive overload [13]. If harm ensues, standard malpractice frameworks may not adequately capture the contributory role of the LLM, and existing tort law offers little clarity on LLM-influenced negligence [13].

Therefore, clinicians must retain active interpretive control over LLM-generated content. The impacts of generative AI in primary care are profound, but without institutional safeguards, legal reform, and ethical clarity, its integration can obscure medical responsibility [14, 15]. Ethical integration requires that outputs be treated as unvalidated suggestions – not surrogate reasoning. Embedding LLMs into clinical workflows without concurrent safeguards for accountability risks not only legal liability but also professional disempowerment [12, 14]. The clinician must remain the ultimate interpreter of clinical truth, regardless of whether that truth originates from human reasoning or LLM-generated algorithmic synthesis.

3. Confidentiality and trust

"Can I Trust the LLM with My Patient's Secrets?"

Primary care is grounded in trust, with confidentiality serving as a cornerstone of the physician-patient relationship. The integration of LLMs into clinical environments raises serious ethical concerns about the security of sensitive health data [16]. Unlike traditional software tools, LLMs operate in ways that make it difficult to guarantee data boundaries. Model outputs may reflect, store, or infer protected health information (PHI) in ways that are not transparent to the end user [16].

Current implementations of LLMs in healthcare often rely on cloud-based APIs managed by third-party vendors. When clinicians input identifiable or clinically sensitive information into these systems – whether for documentation, summarization, or patient communication – the data traverses insecure external networks to external servers for processing. Although many vendors claim to anonymize or secure this information, recent disclosures reveal that LLMs can retain and inadvertently regurgitate data fragments from previous inputs, including personal identifiers, posing significant risks to confidentiality [17, 18].

This technical vulnerability is compounded by regulatory ambiguity. In the United States, HIPAA compliance frameworks were established before the advent of the LLM era. Questions remain about whether LLMs operated by non-covered entities qualify as business associates, and whether their training, fine-tuning, or caching mechanisms are compatible with existing privacy mandates [16, 19]. Furthermore, when patients independently use public-facing LLMs for health queries, those interactions fall entirely outside HIPAA protections and, thus, beyond the reach of clinical oversight or informed consent.

Trust erosion is not only a legal issue but also a relational one. Patients may reasonably question whether LLM-augmented clinical notes or chatbot interactions compromise their privacy. Studies reveal that patient trust in LLM-mediated care declines when clinicians are unable or unwilling to explain how their data is used, stored, or potentially leveraged for model training [20, 21]. A clinician who cannot confidently explain where a patient's data goes or how it might be used undermines the fiduciary basis of care [20]. In primary care settings, where longitudinal relationships and trust hinge on disclosure, perceived breaches or data misuse may cause lasting harm and have durable effects [21].

Thus, any implementation of LLMs in clinical workflows must be accompanied by explicit data governance protocols. These should include limits on identifiable input, strict audit trails, model-use boundaries, and informed consent where applicable. Until these protections are formalized, the ethical imperative remains non-negotiable but straightforward: patient secrets must not become model fodder.

4. Erosion of clinical thinking

"Will LLMs Atrophy My Clinical Skills?"

LLMs provide powerful cognitive support by generating differential diagnoses, treatment plans, and documentation in real-time. However, their utility as clinical extenders comes with a potential cost: erosion of the clinician's diagnostic reasoning [22, 23]. In primary care, where uncertainty is the norm and presentations often lack pathognomonic clarity, cognitive vigilance is critical. The routine deferral of foundational clinical thinking to LLMs may gradually displace active clinical reasoning with passive acceptance of LLM-generated suggestions.

This hazard is not hypothetical. Analogous phenomena have been documented in aviation and radiology, where over-reliance on decision-support systems has led to skill degradation – a phenomenon termed "automation bias" [22, 23]. LLMs deliver authoritative, confident-sounding suggestions despite the underlying mechanism being purely statistical. In the context of medicine, clinicians exposed to LLMs may unconsciously accept well-framed but fundamentally flawed suggestions, even when these suggestions conflict with clinical findings and knowledge [22, 23]. This anchoring effect is hazardous in primary care, where diagnosis often requires pattern recognition over time and contextual inference unavailable to the model.

Moreover, LLMs introduce a cognitive asymmetry: their fluency and confidence can mask their underlying lack of understanding. LLMs are text predictors trained to mimic coherence, which can obscure the fact that the model lacks an accurate understanding or access to patient-specific context [24]. When these outputs are accepted uncritically, the clinician risks substituting statistical mimicry for mechanistic reasoning.

The implications for medical education are equally concerning. Trainees increasingly encounter LLMs as clinical resources, potentially shaping epistemic habits that prioritize information retrieval over diagnostic synthesis, thus preventing the development of foundational skills [22, 24]. If differential construction becomes outsourced, the iterative process of refining diagnostic hypotheses through active synthesis, comparison, and testing may atrophy [23, 24]. In this sense, LLMs could function not as knowledge extenders but as cognitive substitutes – eroding the very competencies they are meant to support.

To mitigate this risk, clinicians must preserve diagnostic authorship. This requires deliberate friction in the use of LLM outputs: pausing to question, verify, and reinterpret rather than accepting suggestions at face value [24]. Documentation generated by LLMs should be treated as a draft – not a diagnostic endpoint – and must be critically edited to reflect the physician's reasoning process [24]. The long-term integrity of clinical judgment depends not on resisting technology but on integrating it without surrendering cognitive agency.

5. The physician-patient relationship in the LLM era

"Does My Patient Want Me or the Machine?"

Empathy is not ancillary in primary care; it is essential to effective therapy. A physician's ability to engage, actively listen, and emotionally respond to their patient is not merely an interpersonal skill but rather a key tenet of effective healing. It promotes adherence, reduces diagnostic error, and directly improves clinical outcomes. Yet LLMs, now embedded in clinical communication tools, have introduced a new variable: simulated empathy [25]. These models generate seemingly compassionate responses through syntactically tailored phrases, contextual memory, and reflective language [25]. These capabilities raise foundational questions about the nature of the therapeutic alliance. If patients feel heard and understood by a model, what remains uniquely human in the clinician's role?

Recent studies have revealed that patients often rate LLM-generated responses as more empathetic and easier to understand than those provided by physicians, particularly in asynchronous messaging or decision-aid scenarios [26]. This observation not only reflects the persuasive fluency of generative text but also highlights the system-level limitations – time, emotional fatigue, documentation burdens, and volume – that pose significant barriers to sustained real-time human empathy in practice [27]. As a result, AI-mediated empathy can be experienced as more consistent, more immediate, and, in some cases, more emotionally validating.

However, the ethical risk lies in the mismatch between emotional resonance and actual relational presence that arises from the erosion of relational accountability when a physician's core interpersonal responsibilities are delegated to a computational model [26]. LLMs do not possess internal states, moral commitments, or memory beyond session context (unless artificially engineered) [27]. Their empathy is computationally constructed from learned linguistic patterns rather than being based on affective presence. Patients using LLMs may feel heard and emotionally validated, while the system's response is unaware, unfeeling, and uninterested; there is no memory continuity beyond the chat encounter [26]. When patients receive emotionally resonant messages from a non-sentient model, the resulting relationship is asymmetrical and potentially deceptive [25]. This misalignment may erode informed consent, especially if the model's non-human status is unclear.

Further, reliance on LLMs for relational labor may change physician behavior. In high-volume practices, LLMs are increasingly proposed as front-line communicators for delivering lab results, routine counseling, and even diagnostic explanations [26]. Using an LLM as a substitute rather than a supplement may cause physicians to offload core obligations – presence, accountability, and moral responsibility – resulting in depersonalized care [27]. Delegating these interactions risks narrowing the clinician's role to technical oversight, thereby commodifying what was once a core dimension of healing: presence [27].

Physicians must therefore reassert the ethical centrality of relational labor. While LLMs can augment communication, they cannot replace the embodied moral presence that undergirds trust [25]. Transparency is essential – patients must know when they are interacting with a machine. A recent review found that patient trust in LLMs was highest when a physician was present, mediating communication, and lowest when the LLM was used as a substitute for a human moderator [28]. Thus, further proof is provided that the use of LLMs in patient communication should be additive, not substitutive: enhancing access or efficiency without replacing the bidirectional, meaning-making dialog that defines human care [25, 28].

In this LLM era, the clinician's role may evolve – but it cannot be reduced. The therapeutic value of being known, remembered, and cared for cannot be emulated by even the most linguistically adept machine [25].

6. Counseling patients about LLM therapists

"My Patient Is Using LLM as a Therapist - What Now?"

In under-resourced settings, or among patients facing financial, geographic, or cultural barriers to mental health care, LLM-based tools are increasingly used as informal therapists [29]. Accessible through mobile devices, chat interfaces, or integrated health apps, LLMs offer patients a semblance of listening, reflection, and even problem-solving [28]. This emergent phenomenon introduces a complex ethical terrain for primary care clinicians, who often serve as the default mental health providers for their patients.

LLMs can produce therapeutic-sounding responses that emulate techniques from cognitive behavioral therapy, motivational interviewing, or psychodynamic reflection [29]. Yet, they are not trained mental health professionals, nor are they capable of clinical assessment, emotional attunement, or crisis intervention. LLMs create the illusion of professional support when none exists [29]. Patients who rely on LLMs for psychological support may unknowingly receive content that is unvalidated, non-specific, or even harmful in the context of suicidality, trauma, or psychosis [29].

Moreover, these interactions occur outside any formal clinical setting. There is no therapeutic contract, no confidentiality in the traditional sense, and no legal or ethical framework governing the exchange [16]. Data shared with LLM platforms may be stored, monetized, or repurposed without the patient's awareness [14, 16]. Some models lack guardrails to prevent the creation of suggestive or misleading statements, especially in emotionally charged contexts. In this way, LLMs can act as pseudo-clinicians without bearing any of the fiduciary, legal, or ethical obligations of care.

Clinicians must be prepared to acknowledge and address LLM-integrated care [30]. They must recognize that patients may seek LLM-based support due to accessibility barriers, stigma, or prior negative experiences with traditional healthcare. In contrast, others may engage due to a lack of awareness that the tool is non-human or unregulated [30]. Validation is essential. Patients should not be shamed or dismissed for seeking support where it is available. Physicians should assess patients' perceived benefits and risks associated with LLM usage and, if necessary, clarify the scope and limitations of LLM use [30]. Moreover, physicians should guide patients to safer alternatives, such as support group networks and teletherapy. Another option may be to utilize a mixed-use model, where clinicians use LLM as care supplementation for early reflections, while decisions involve face-to-face shared decision-making [30]. Most importantly, physicians must engage in shared follow-up not only to establish physical presence and build patient rapport but also to assess the emotional impacts of LLM use, identify adverse effects of LLM usage, and clarify any concerns or questions that may arise from patient use [29, 30].

Ethically, the clinician's role is twofold: to validate the patient's pursuit of support while clarifying the limitations and potential harms of LLM-based therapy [29]. This conversation should be approached with neutrality and framed within the broader commitment to safety, privacy, and continuity of care [30]. Where appropriate, referrals should be made to qualified human providers, but the clinician must recognize that LLM-based support may persist regardless [30]. The goal is not to eliminate its use, but to contextualize it – and ensure it occurs within a framework of informed awareness. Regardless of whether future LLMs demonstrate high diagnostic and therapeutic efficacy, profound ethical issues of trust, liability, and human relational presence remain.

7. Conclusion

The integration of large language models into primary care is not a distant prospect – it is an active transformation unfolding in clinical practice. These systems offer undeniable efficiencies in documentation, diagnostics, and communication [31]. Yet, these benefits also introduce profound ethical hazards that are distinctively shaped by the nature of frontline medicine, including time constraints, ambiguous symptoms, emotional fatigue, and relational continuity dilemmas, which abstract AI ethics frameworks do not encounter [15, 20, 32].

This chapter outlines several emergent hazards, including liability displacement, confidentiality risks, cognitive offloading, empathy simulation, and the rise of LLM-as-therapist dynamics. Across these domains, one constant remains: the clinician is the final ethical filter [25]. Regardless of how persuasive, efficient, or accurate LLMs appear, their outputs require physician judgment, skepticism, and contextualization [33].

Therefore, ethical practice in the LLM era demands more than technical competence [27]. Physicians must remain critical of well-written but potentially flawed LLM outputs, vigilant in protecting privacy, and unapologetic in defending the relational core of care [27]. Practical skepticism means questioning confident-sounding LLM outputs, especially when they conflict with clinical intuition or patient-specific context. Accountability must adapt to the growing role of LLMs, yet medicine is an inherently human duty that cannot be abdicated to a machine [34].

LLMs and generative AI models will continue to evolve, further embedding into electronic health records, patient portals, and clinical workflows, reshaping the clinical landscape. However, the ethical center of medicine – its accountability, empathy, and clinical reasoning – must not be outsourced. In the presence of transformative technology, the task is not to retreat but to remain: fully present, fully responsible, and fully human. **Table 1** summarizes these principles into actionable recommendations for clinical practice.

Ethical Domain	Core Principle	Practical Actions
Liability & Clinical Judgment	Maintain diagnostic authorship	• Treat LLM outputs as unvalidated suggestions. • Pause to question and verify before accepting. • Document your reasoning process, not just the LLM output. • Never delegate final decisions to the LLM.
Confidentiality & Trust	Protect patient data boundaries	• Use only HIPAA-compliant, on-premises LLM tools whenever possible. • Avoid inputting identifiable information into cloud-based LLMs. • Establish clear data governance protocols. • Inform patients about the use of LLM and data.
Clinical Reasoning	Preserve cognitive vigilance	• Use LLMs as a supplement, not a substitute for thinking. • Deliberately question LLM-generated differentials • Edit LLM documentation to reflect your reasoning. • Maintain diagnostic skills through active practice.
Physician-Patient Relationship	Prioritize authentic human connection	• Be transparent about LLM involvement in communication. • Use LLM to enhance, not replace personal interaction. • Preserve time for direct patient engagement. • Clarify when patients are interacting with an LLM versus a human.
Patient AI Use	Validate and guide safely	• Ask non-judgmentally about patient LLM use. • Clarify limitations and risks of LLM therapy. • Provide alternative resources when appropriate. • Follow up on the emotional impacts of LLM interactions

Ethical Domain	Core Principle	Practical Actions
General Principles (All Domains)	Core principles for all domains	• Transparency: Always disclose LLM involvement to patients. • Accountability: Physicians remain fully responsible for all clinical decisions. • Critical Evaluation: Question LLM outputs rather than accepting them uncritically. • Human-Centered Care: Preserve the relational core of medicine • Continuous Learning: Stay informed about LLM capabilities and limitations.

Table 1.
Key ethical recommendations for LLM use in primary care.

Acknowledgments

The authors acknowledge support from the Department of Family Medicine at the University of Washington and the Department of Medical Education and Clinical Sciences at Washington State University. The authors thank all clinical colleagues who offered case insights and discussions during the preparation of this chapter.

Conflict of interest

The authors declare no conflicts of interest

Author details

Michelle Lu[1], Justin J. Gillette[2] and Thomas F. Heston[2*]

1 School of Medicine, University of Washington, Seattle, Washington, USA

2 Elson S. Floyd College of Medicine, Washington State University, Spokane, Washington, United States of America

*Address all correspondence to: theston@uw.edu

References

[1] Amann J, Blasimme A, Vayena E, Frey D, Madai VI. Precise4Q consortium. Explainability for artificial intelligence in healthcare: A multidisciplinary perspective. BMC Medical Informatics and Decision Making. 2020;**20**(1):310

[2] Li H, Moon JT, Purkayastha S, Celi LA, Trivedi H, Gichoya JW. Ethics of large language models in medicine and medical research. The Lancet Digital Health. 2023;**5**(6):e333–5

[3] Currie GM, Hawk KE, Rohren EM. Generative artificial intelligence biases, limitations and risks in nuclear medicine: An argument for appropriate use framework and recommendations. Seminars in Nuclear Medicine. 2024;**55**:423–436

[4] Heston TF. Safety of large language models in addressing depression. Cureus. 2023;**15**(12):e50729

[5] Ayers JW, Poliak A, Dredze M, Leas EC, Zhu Z, Kelley JB, et al. Comparing physician and artificial intelligence chatbot responses to patient questions posted to a public social media forum. JAMA Internal Medicine 2023;**183**:589–596

[6] Gabison GA, Xian RP. Inherent and emergent liability issues in LLM-based agentic systems: A principal-agent perspective. In: Proceedings of the 1st Workshop for Research on Agent Language Models (REALM 2025). Stroudsburg, PA, USA: Association for Computational Linguistics; 2025. p. 109–130

[7] Hao Y, Qiu Z, Holmes J, Löckenhoff CE, Liu W, Ghassemi M, et al. Large language model integrations in cancer decision-making: A systematic review and meta-analysis. NPJ Digital Medicine 2025;**8**:450

[8] Mesinovic M, Watkinson P, Zhu T. Explainability in the age of large language models for healthcare. Communications Engineering. 2025;**4**(1):128

[9] Gerke S, Minssen T, Cohen G. Artificial Intelligence in Healthcare. In: Bohr A, Memarzadeh K, eds. Chapter 12 - Ethical and legal challenges of artificial intelligence-driven healthcare. Academic Press; 2020. p. 295–336. DOI: 10.1016/B978-0-12-818438-7.00012-5

[10] Naik N, Hameed BMZ, Shetty DK, Swain D, Shah M, Paul R, et al. Legal and ethical consideration in artificial intelligence in healthcare: Who takes responsibility? Frontiers in Surgery. 2022;**9**:862322. DOI: 10.3389/fsurg.2022.862322

[11] Lee B, Naftalovich R, Ali S, Chaudhry FA, Tewfik GL. Liability exposure of clinicians in Artificial Intelligence-Driven healthcare. Biomedical Instrumentation & Technology. 2024;**58**(2):39–42

[12] Warraich HJ, Tazbaz T, Califf RM. FDA perspective on the regulation of artificial intelligence in health care and biomedicine. JAMA. 2025;**333**(3): 241–247

[13] Mennella C, Maniscalco U, De Pietro G, Esposito M. Ethical and regulatory challenges of AI technologies in healthcare: A narrative review. Heliyon. 2024;**10**(4):e26297

[14] Price IIWN, Gerke S, Cohen IG. Liability for use of artificial intelligence in medicine. In: Solaiman B, Cohen IG, editors. Research Handbook on Health, AI and the Law. Cheltenham, UK: Edward Elgar Publishing Ltd; 2024. p. 150–166

[15] Habli I, Lawton T, Porter Z. Artificial intelligence in health care: Accountability and safety. Bulletin of the World Health Organization. 2020;**98**(4):251–256

[16] Murdoch B. Privacy and artificial intelligence: Challenges for protecting health information in a new era. BMC Medical Ethics. 2021;**22**(1):122

[17] Dennstädt F, Hastings J, Putora PM, Schmerder M, Cihoric N. Implementing large language models in healthcare while balancing control, collaboration, costs and security. Npj Digital Medicine. 2025;**8**(1):143

[18] Privacy International. Large language models and data protection [Internet]. Privacy International. 2024. Available from: https://privacyinternational.org/explainer/5353/large-language-models-and-data-protection [Accessed: 2025-August-19]

[19] Ziller A, Mueller TT, Stieger S, Feiner LF, Brandt J, Braren R, et al. Reconciling privacy and accuracy in AI for medical imaging. Nature Machine Intelligence 2024;**6**:764–774

[20] Zondag AGM, Rozestraten R, Grimmelikhuijsen SG, Jongsma KR, van Solinge WW, Bots ML, et al. The effect of Artificial Intelligence on patient-physician trust: Cross-sectional vignette study. Journal of Medical Internet Research. 2024;**26**: e50853

[21] Esmaeilzadeh P, Mirzaei T, Dharanikota S. Patients' perceptions toward Human-Artificial Intelligence interaction in health care: Experimental study. Journal of Medical Internet Research. 2021;**23**(11):e25856

[22] Zhai C, Wibowo S, Li LD. The effects of over-reliance on AI dialogue systems on students' cognitive abilities: A systematic review. Smart Learning Environments. 2024;**11**(1):28

[23] Jones N. Does using ChatGPT change your brain activity? Study Sparks debate. Nature. 2025;**643** (8070):15–16

[24] Choudhury A, Chaudhry Z. Large language models and user trust: Consequence of Self-Referential learning loop and the deskilling of health care professionals. Journal of Medical Internet Research. 2024;**26**:e56764

[25] Montemayor C, Halpern J, Fairweather A. In principle obstacles for empathic AI: Why we can't replace human empathy in healthcare. AI & Society. 2022;**37**(4):1353–1359

[26] Karoulla E, Matragkas N, Islam SU, Epiphaniou G. Challenges and risks of using synthetic data for AI-Driven healthcare applications. Studies in Health Technology and Informatics. 2025;**328**:81–85

[27] Allen MR, Webb S, Mandvi A, Frieden M, Tai-Seale M, Kallenberg G. Navigating the doctor-patient-AI relationship - a mixed-methods study of physician attitudes toward artificial intelligence in primary care. BMC Primary Care. 2024;**25**(1):42

[28] Steerling E, Siira E, Nilsen P, Svedberg P, Nygren J. Implementing AI

in healthcare-the relevance of trust: A scoping review. Frontiers in Health Services. 2023;**3**:1211150

[29] Coghlan S, Leins K, Sheldrick S, Cheong M, Gooding P, D'Alfonso S. To chat or bot to chat: Ethical issues with using chatbots in mental health. Digital Health. 2023;**9**:20552076231183542

[30] Schiff D, Borenstein J. How should clinicians communicate with patients about the roles of artificially intelligent team members? AMA Journal of Ethics. 2019;**21**(2):E138–145

[31] Sallam M. Chatgpt utility in healthcare education, research, and practice: Systematic review on the promising perspectives and valid concerns. Healthcare (Basel). 2023;**11**(6):887

[32] Cestonaro C, Delicati A, Marcante B, Caenazzo L, Tozzo P. Defining medical liability when artificial intelligence is applied on diagnostic algorithms: A systematic review. Frontiers in Medicine (Lausanne). 2023;**10**:1305756

[33] Lambert SI, Madi M, Sopka S, Lenes A, Stange H, Buszello C-P, et al. An integrative review on the acceptance of artificial intelligence among healthcare professionals in hospitals. NPJ Digital Medicine 2023;**6**:111

[34] Price WN, Cohen IG. Privacy in the age of medical big data. Nature Medicine. 2019;**25**(1):37–43

Chapter 7

Perspective Chapter: Lines, Lives, and Lessons – What Dialysis Teaches Us about the Role of Ethics and Sustainability in Modern Medicine

Ana Mateus, Pedro Ponce and Ivo Laranjinha

Abstract

In this chapter, the clinical scenario of a very frail elderly patient about to start dialysis is used to show how dialysis – a treatment that was long ago considered exceptional and ethically controversial – has become a routine procedure, often applied without adequate ethical reflection. Several aspects are analysed, such as the evolution of clinical limits, bedside decisions, environmental impact, and system-level responsibility. Starting from a main case, each section develops each of the major challenges faced by modern nephrology. This paper is intended for all healthcare professionals who care for patients with kidney disease and has been written as a perspective narrative.

Keywords: dialysis ethics, end-of-life care, shared decision-making, sustainability, health systems

1. Introduction

The use of dialysis has witnessed tremendous development in recent decades, from being a unique and ethically problematic treatment to a more routine and accepted form of therapy. With dialysis being more widely available, it has become more commonly used in elderly and vulnerable patients, thereby giving rise to ethical concerns about its use in such a patient group. In this chapter, the ethical issues involved in dialysis will be discussed using the case study of an 84-year-old female patient referred to as Mrs. A and will be used to illustrate the main ethical issues involved in dialysis therapy. In this case study, it will be discussed how decisions regarding dialysis therapy must be made in accordance with ethical principles such as autonomy, beneficence, non-maleficence, and justice not only from the patient's perspective but also from a broader healthcare and environmental perspective. In this case study, two different care pathways will be discussed to illustrate the importance of shared decision-making and the role that palliative care models must be incorporated in such decisions. In this case study, it will also be discussed how healthcare professionals must manage such ethical decisions and dilemmas and the legal and environmental issues that must be addressed in such a patient group.

Finally, it will be highlighted that in modern-day nephrology, it is important that a way be found to integrate technological advancements with patient dignity and respect for our planet's future and that dialysis therapy is no longer used as a routine form of therapy but must be incorporated in accordance with patient values and goals in therapy and that this requires ethical consideration at each step in a patient's journey from chronic renal disease to acute crisis situations.

2. Clinical Case Report: Mrs. A – Two pathways, two different results

Mrs. A is an 84-year-old woman who lives with her daughter in a semi-rural community. She has a long history of diabetes, hypertension, end-stage heart failure, and stage 4 chronic kidney disease (baseline estimated glomerular filtration rate of approximately 25 ml/min). Over the past year, she suffered a dramatic decline: she became more dependent, refused to leave the house, needed help with feeding and caring for herself, and experienced significant weight loss. She has not been followed by a nephrologist, but previous laboratory tests revealed a progressive worsening of her renal function. Her Canadian Frailty Scale (CFS) score was 7 (severe frailty), and her Palliative Performance Scale (PPS) was 50%, indicating a poor prognosis.

2.1 Scenario 1 – A beginning lacking strategic planning

Mrs. A came to the emergency department with dyspnoea, peripheral oedema, and fatigue. She was fluid-overloaded and oliguric, and blood tests showed severe renal impairment (creatinine 7.2 mg/dL, urea 230 mg/dL), hyperkalaemia ($K+$ 6.4 mmol/L), and metabolic acidosis. She continued to be overloaded despite intravenous diuretics. There was no advance care directive. Her daughter remembered her mother's prior expressions against aggressive treatment, but her son insisted: '*We will do everything. This is not the time to stop.*'

In the acute-on-chronic kidney injury cases, dialysis was initiated through a central venous catheter. Despite hemodynamic stabilization, Mrs. A did not regain appetite or independence. The demanding thrice-weekly 120-km round trips to the dialysis center proved exhausting, and within three weeks, she began refusing further sessions. Her daughter said, '*I don't think she would have wanted this.*' The attending medical team started discussions about the withdrawal of dialysis treatment.

Looking back on the case, one of the junior nephrologists on the team commented: '*We have moved quickly because we could. But should we have acted that way? In an overburdened system with scarce resources and dialysis being a treatment materially challenging and ethically complex, are we making decisions in line with the patient's life and wishes, or are we being motivated by less important values?*'

2.2 Scenario 2 – Another way

In a second approach, when Mrs. A arrived with acute decompensation and alarming laboratory results, the admission team, in agreement with the nephrology team, took some time to allow for shared decision-making before deciding whether to start dialysis. A family meeting was held, including her son and daughter, the nephrologist, the palliative care consultant, and the nursing team. The doctors discussed the patient's clinical trajectory, her prognosis, and the possible benefits and burdens of dialysis in the context of her frailty.

The daughter reminded her mother of her earlier declarations opposing the extension of life through mechanical means. The son, who had initially supported maximal medical treatment, changed his view after weighing the small anticipated gains and the high treatment burden. The family reached a consensus to adopt a conservative management approach focused on comfort, symptom palliation, and care within the home setting. Changes were made to increase the use of diuretics, a low-protein diet was started, and advance care planning was completed, including issuing a do-not-dialysis order. Community palliative care services were activated to ensure ongoing follow-up and support prior to Mrs. A's discharge home.

3. Subchapter 1: Thresholds and boundaries in dialysis ethics

3.1 From exception to routine

When it first appeared in the mid-20th century, dialysis was a new and controversial treatment. Access was limited, options were restricted, and starting dialysis most of the time involved a moral choice: why should this patient and not that one have the chance to prolong his life? Those choices were often painful and mostly fatal [1].

Today, in all but a few low-income countries, dialysis is common, the technology is standardized, and when biochemical markers reach certain levels, starting a patient on treatment is often an automatic response [2–4]. The pendulum has swung from not having enough to having too much, but along with the excess has come the slow decline of moral thinking. Dialysis is no longer a remarkable treatment; it is simply what we do when the kidneys fail, and it remains the only life-prolonging treatment universally covered by public insurance [5].

For some time, the age of the patient discreetly influenced access to hemodialysis, but this practice was abandoned following strong criticism of age discrimination [6, 7].

In recent decades, the demographic profile of patients with end-stage kidney disease (ESKD) has changed dramatically. With increased life expectancy and the consequent aging of populations, dialysis patients are increasingly elderly and frail, displaying multiple comorbidities and representing the fastest-growing demographic group in dialysis treatment. Therefore, it is a priority to carefully consider, for each patient, the real benefit and possible burden of dialysis, keeping in mind that any decisions have not only medical implications but also ethical, legal, and ecological ones [8–10].

The increase in the number of elderly and frail dialysis patients raises crucial ethical questions: Are we really helping patients? Are we doing what patients want? Are we avoiding undue harm? These questions reflect the fundamental principles of medical ethics – justice, autonomy, beneficence, and non-maleficence – that have guided decision-making from Hippocratic practice to contemporary clinical care [11–13].

In scenario 1, the central ethical dilemma is whether the treatment aligns with the patient's values, care goals, and preferences. This represents a shift from the initial focus on biochemical goals to a broader moral challenge of determining what constitutes appropriate and meaningful treatment. This is particularly difficult when the patient has lost cognitive function and can no longer participate in decision-making. In such situations, physicians must rely on family members' accounts of the patient.

Frailty is a moral concept for Mrs. A, not just a clinical term. It is an indicator of a higher mortality rate, a significantly faster functional decline over time, a lower quality of life, and a greater likelihood of living in a nursing home. These are burdens that dialysis is likely to exacerbate [14]. Additionally, patients who initiate dialysis with a Clinical Frailty Scale score of five or higher experience shorter survival rates and increased hospitalisations[15].

As explained in Subchapter 2, it might be difficult to distinguish between futility and treatment. When we are ready to see this narrow line before the crucial moment, when patients and their families may reflect and rationalise without the stress of time running out in the emergency department, it becomes clearer.

3.2 Ethics of unplanned dialysis in frail patients

Decision-making about the initiation, suspension, and withdrawal of dialysis is complex and, ideally, occurs over time in the context of the therapeutic relationship between the patient and healthcare professional, with early involvement of the family.

In the case of unplanned dialysis for frail patients without decision-making capacity, the most relevant ethical principle is that of autonomy. Respecting autonomy requires that treatment decisions align with the patient's individual preferences and values. However, when the patient cannot express such preferences, it becomes especially challenging to preserve the integrity of their autonomy.

Family members are commonly asked to act as the patient's spokesperson, but this can impose emotional and moral burdens. They may feel coerced, concerned that refusing dialysis could be perceived as killing the patient, even if it is in accordance with what the patient would have wanted. This emphasises the value of advance care planning and explicit documentation of the patient's wishes. If this does not exist, the clinical team needs to support families by providing clear and honest information, avoiding an imposed decision, and rather adopting a solution aligned with the patient's values and previously expressed interests.

3.3 The lack of palliative care trainees in nephrology

Starting dialysis is a medical and ethical decision for every patient, but it is particularly important for older or frail individuals. Offering haemodialysis (HD) indiscriminately has led to many frail elderly patients being harmed by overly aggressive treatment near the end-of-life (EOL), violating the principle of non-maleficence. Moreover, dialysis patients are also more likely to undergo aggressive interventions in their last month and die in hospitals [16], despite evidence that most patients would prefer to die at home or in hospice [17]. This suggests that patients are often unprepared for EOL, partly because nephrologists feel unprepared to provide such care [18, 19].

Ethics, communication, and EOL care training are not always a part of nephrology training around the world, even though there is robust evidence recommending the introduction of level 2 palliative care training and skills development in nephrology to address those gaps [19–23].

Bringing ethics into nephrology training means making it normal to talk about ending as much as starting, conservative treatment as a reasonable choice, and the environmental impact of what we do. It is about building organizational cultures that support doctors in making patient-centered, resource-conscious choices, even when those choices mean 'doing less'.

These thresholds and planning failures lead us into the next discussion: how to define the line when dialysis crosses into futility, as well as how to navigate the moral distress that is triggered by such decisions, as will be explored in the subchapter 2.

4. Subchapter 2: Between futility and moral distress – Human aspects of medical decision-making

Historically, in 1991, the Institute of Medicine (IOM) Committee responsible for the study of the Medicare end-stage renal disease highlighted the need for a clinical practice guideline 'aiming to evaluate patients for whom the burdens of renal replacement treatment may substantially outweigh the benefits' [24].

Following the IOM recommendation, a first shared decision-making guideline was published, providing clinicians, patients, and families with relevant information about the benefits and burdens of dialysis for patients displaying different types of medical conditions [25].

However, it was recognized that there are some limits to the process: 'informed consent does not mean that patients can insist upon anything they want'; patients may only choose among medically accepted and available options that are believed to promote the patient's welfare [26].

4.1 Lessons from Mrs. A

Scenario I: We learn from this short summary that she was increasingly dependent, refusing to leave her home, with a high frailty score and ongoing cognitive decline. Although family members, as quite often happens, remember hearing Mrs. A discuss or make clear statements of her wishes about EOL care, when the time comes, the consensus generated at the last minute is to go ahead with the full treatment she so clearly refused.

We usually trust that advance care planning (ACP) is a reassurance that the autonomy of all our patients, including those who lost their decision-making capacity long before their demise, will be respected once confronted with difficult end-of-life decisions [27, 28].

However, more recent evidence suggests that having issued an ACP does not, in and of itself, guarantee that those same patients will have a meaningful discussion with their healthcare proxies or that its documentation will improve end-of-life care, avoiding futile hospitalizations, surgery, or intensive care unit admissions [29, 30].

The answer may be to incentivise patients to rely on the appointment of a trusted surrogate decision-maker while still in control of their lives, to keep him always updated on one's goals, fears, and major concerns, and "educate" him on the several scenarios he may soon have to face, as well as the ritual of participation in shared decision-making with the attending physician.

Again, this reliance on the health care proxy to improve EOL care and its superiority compared to a standard ACP needs to be demonstrated.

Scenario II: Mrs. A arrived at the last-minute decision exactly in the same situation as scenario I. The difference was that maybe her daughter was better informed and therefore more outspoken, giving full credit and relevance to what she believed were the wishes of her mother, and a better-educated team was willing to hold, on short notice, a family meeting to decide on EOL care. Once the decision was taken to proceed with conservative treatment, palliative care was involved. However, in case there was a nephrologist and a renal nurse in the team, they should be able to provide basic palliative and comfort care and never abandon the case.

Treatment choices near the EOL are not simple, consistent, logical, linear, or predictable, but are complex, uncertain, emotionally laden, and fluid. Patients' preferences are rarely static and are influenced by age, physical and cognitive function, culture, family preferences, clinical advice, financial resources, and perceived caregiver burden, all of which change over time. Surrogates find it difficult to extrapolate treatment decisions in the present from hypothetical discussions with patients that occurred in the past, overcome their own preferences and emotions, or challenge physicians who recommend different treatments. When a decision must be made, prior directives are often absent, poorly documented, or either so prescriptive or so vague that they can hardly be used on patients' behalf.

Therefore, although the ethical aspects of clinical decisions are now well characterized and discussed at length, individual cases continue to present us with very difficult and distressing choices. Physicians must always be prepared for the possibility that patient preferences may change over time due to new events. Additionally, some patients or family members may never be able to decide or express their preferences. Some may prefer to receive limited or no information and delegate decision-making to others – in our Portuguese experience, mainly their attending physicians [31].

4.2 Medical futility

The term 'medical futility' refers to excessive medical intervention (both in terms of medical effort and financial resources) that is unlikely to improve the patient's final clinical outcome. The risk of futility is almost always present in everyday medical practice. The question is: who decides whether a treatment is futile or not, and is it futile for the patient or for the payer?

A few disturbing facts: *(i)* In a Canadian study, 61% of patients regretted commencing dialysis, 52% of them reported that it was their physician's wish, and in 14%, it was their family's wish [32]. *(ii)* Elderly patients on hemodialysis report that their entire day is often taken up traveling to and from the dialysis unit and undergoing the treatment itself. Dialysis prolongs the survival of elderly patients with ESRD who have significant comorbidities by approximately 2 years, but patients who choose not to start dialysis may survive for a similar period without an increase in the number of hospital admissions [33].

In the special group of nursing home residents, within the first year after the initiation of dialysis, 58% of all the residents had died, 29% experienced a decrease in functional status, which was maintained in only 13%, and 30% abandoned dialysis due to major physical or cognitive deterioration [14].

According to recent data from the United States Renal Data System (USRDS), 1 in every 4 patients starting dialysis is over 75. Moreover, they have a higher prevalence of comorbidities and geriatric syndromes, which dramatically reduce their life expectancy and impair their informed decision-making capability [34, 35].

While it may seem adequate to refuse therapies potentially futile for some patients, thereby preserving precious resources for patients with more opportunities to ameliorate their health, this kind of rationale does not ensure fair health care, nor better medical results or care [36].

4.3 Autonomy and its limitations

The initiation of dialysis assumes the appropriate provision of informed consent. Ideally, such a process begins as a part of ACP done long before a person is faced with a decision about initiating or not initiating a renal replacement treatment (RRT).

The importance of ACP is highlighted by the high rates of dialysis discontinuation, which is the second leading cause of death after cardiovascular disease and accounts for a quarter of deaths among dialysis patients [37].

Informed consent stems from the right to privacy, involves the expression of self-determination and independence, and is based on the ethical principle of autonomy.

More than simply signing a form, it represents a process of communication between doctor and patient that establishes a relationship of trust and allows the patient to decide whether to undergo medical intervention.

The physician who obtains consent from the patient or their family does not have to present all available treatment options. Their professional responsibility, in accordance with the shared decision-making guidelines, is only to exercise clinical judgement and guide the patient/family through the clinically indicated options, rather than presenting options that are not real options [38].

When discussing informed consent with elderly patients with CKD, it should be made clear that: (*i*) dialysis may not confer a survival advantage over medical treatment; (*ii*) patients may experience no significant functional improvement, or even no improvement at all, with dialysis.

The explanation of treatment options should include: (*i*) available dialysis modalities; (*ii*) not starting dialysis and continuing conservative treatment, including EOL care; (*iii*) a trial period of dialysis of limited duration; (*iv*) discontinuation of dialysis and receipt of EOL care.

It is also a well-known fact that neither attending physicians nor close family members can accurately predict patients' wishes regarding the type and intensity of care they desire in their final months of life, failing to do so in about 50% of cases [39].

Although, in a recent series, 81% of dialysis patients observed had completed a healthcare proxy and living will, of all those with advanced directives, only about half significantly helped in the treatment of patients [40].

A patient's inability to complete a written advance directive or decide about the end of life does not change the standards that their healthcare provider must require of their representatives when making decisions on their behalf. These standards include the patient's previously expressed wishes, surrogate judgement, and best interests.

Therefore, the question remains: How can we give autonomy to those who cannot use it and never impose it on those who want to renounce their right?

In addition, part of this – and, in our opinion, extremely relevant – is the appointment of a healthcare proxy, an agent (substitute) to act on behalf of the patient if they become incompetent. This is the most effective way to ensure that the patient's autonomy will, in fact, be protected, even in cases not mentioned or provided for in the living will. Educating surrogates about why dialysis is no longer an appropriate and useful treatment for a particular patient is critical to helping them represent the patient [41].

Doctors may also face requests from families to withhold information from patients. How can I respect autonomy while honoring the family's request to withhold information that they believe will harm the patient? We should try to understand the family's point of view and be flexible. It is important to explain to the family what the patient would likely want and to propose a negotiated approach on how to clarify with the patient how they want clinical information to be managed – including what they want to know, who should be involved in receiving the information, and when it should be disclosed [42].

4.4 Moral distress in professionals

Several stages of the decision-making process in ethical dilemmas are sources of professional and moral distress, or what has more recently been recognised as burnout. Relevant moments that induce this moral distress include:

i. Physicians are often reluctant to destroy the remaining hope of patients and family members by providing prognostic information.

ii. It is often easier to follow standard treatment protocols than to engage in difficult conversations.

iii. There is persistent uncertainty about what the patient has understood from the information provided, about their real motivations for making a decision, and about the consistency of that decision over time.

iv. Nephrologists generally lack experience in discussing conservative treatment and determining the best time to initiate such conversations. Postponing discussions is, therefore, the most frequent approach.

v. Physicians also have a natural aversion to potential litigation with family members, conflicts with the nephrologist who referred the patient, disappointing the expectations of the administration, or compromising their own personal interests.

vi. Prognostic models are reliable for large populations, but they are not accurate in predicting outcomes for individual patients.

   Prognostic tools should not be applied to deny treatment to an individual patient outside the context in which they were validated, especially without a full understanding of the degree of uncertainty in the estimates obtained.

vii. Finally, patients often want to receive accurate and honest prognostic information while, at the same time, expecting their doctors to remain optimistic about their prognosis.

To ease this distress, we desperately need better training, the removal of economic, legal, and administrative barriers, and easier access to a palliative care specialist for more complex situations.

4.5 Legal implications of our ethical decisions

The definition of a competent patient has key legal implications in the assessment of our ethically guided decisions. The patient considered to be mentally competent and holding decision-making capacity must: (*i*) fully understand the relevant clinical information provided; (*ii*) understand the possible consequences and final outcomes of their clinical situation; (*iii*) understand and distinguish between the different diagnostic and therapeutic options presented; and (*iv*) be able to communicate their decisions and choices [38].

Always be aware that different countries may have different laws and regulations; namely, withdrawing does not always have the same legal value as withholding dialysis. The legal system and medical profession don't always recognize ACP and living wills, and local religion and culture may constitute important hurdles to the application of modern ethics, as depicted in this subchapter.

5. Subchapter 3: The unseen footprint – Environmental ethics in dialysis

The environmental impact of dialysis broadens the concept of responsibility beyond the patient and the clinical environment by considering the sustainability of our clinical decisions for generations to come.

5.1 Environmental effects of dialysis: Water, plastic and use of electricity

Extreme climate events, as well as poor water and air quality, have been associated with kidney diseases progressing rapidly. While being a life-sustaining treatment, dialysis is one of the most resource-consuming (water and energy) and waste-producing medical activities [43].

A standard hemodialysis (HD) session (4-hour treatment, usually thrice a week) uses 380 to 500 liters of tap water, depending on the efficiency of the reverse osmosis (RO), and 10 to 18 kWh of energy per patient [44, 45].

An average patient undergoing in-center HD can generate more than 2 kg of waste per session (390 kg/year, equivalent to the volume produced by an inhabitant in a developed country). One-third of dialysis waste is plastic, namely polyvinyl chloride (PVC) (one of the most environmentally damaging plastics), biohazardous, or pharmaceutical waste, such as lines, dialyzers, bags, syringes, gauze, medications, etc. [43].

The carbon footprint (CFP) of HD, although variable from country to country, is as high as 3 to 10.3 tonnes of CO_2/patient/year[48,49], which is equivalent to driving 37,000 km in an average passenger vehicle. Significant differences in the main contributors to the CFP of HD across countries depend mainly on the energy source (fossil fuels or renewable energy), travel distance to HD facilities, as well as other contextual factors[46].

A dialysis patient generates 7 to 10 times the carbon emissions as compared to an average patient in the UK and Portugal, respectively [47].

Dialysis units significantly contribute to pharmaceutical waste, including unused or expired drugs and drug-containing waste materials. Untreated and even treated wastewater contains pharmaceutical residues that flow into ecosystems, and the impact of most of these drugs remains largely unknown.

5.2 Global expansion of demand for dialysis and environmental cost

Today, an estimated 850 million people worldwide suffer from CKD.

With the progressive aging of the population and the increase in the prevalence of cardiometabolic diseases, together with greater availability of dialysis, there will be a significant increase in the number of RRTs worldwide.

By 2030, it is estimated that the number of people requiring RRT will exceed 5.4 million, with the largest increase in Asia and Africa [48].

In that scenario, HD will become unsustainable in less than a decade.

5.3 Ethical considerations of sustainability and justice between generations

Environmental sustainability of healthcare can present ethical tensions: (i) patients living in developed vs. developing countries; (ii) present vs. future generations; (iii) humankind vs. nature; (iv) global vs. local impact; and (v) individual vs. collective well-being.

Nature should not be viewed as an external resource but rather as our shared and unique home, supporting essential aspects of sustaining our lives as well as the interdependence between human, animal, and environmental health.

Evidence showing that climate change, pollutants, and other environmental stressors are associated with faster progression of chronic kidney disease (CKD) and an increased risk of ESKD highlights the urgent need for advanced environmental sustainability.

A striking example is investing in the prevention of CKD – by avoiding, delaying, or minimizing progression to ESKD. However, the effects of prevention take time, and our societies are still not thinking about healthcare in the most rational or effective way [49].

Introducing environmental sustainability into healthcare creates an ethical dilemma: saving lives or restoring health today while preserving natural resources for future generations.

HD alternatives, such as conservative treatment of ESKD, can be more appropriate for the patient and aligned with family expectations while offering a significantly lower CFP.

5.4 Greener technologies and approaches

New technologies and approaches have been developed to reduce the CFP of HD treatments – some based on truly innovative solutions.

To reduce water usage, it is possible to implement more efficient treatment systems or reutilise wastewater from dialysis.

Furthermore, dialysis effluent with large concentrations of nutrients can be used in gardening or agriculture. Microbial and antibiotic contamination data are limited, and more investigations are needed to generalize its use.

Dialysate effluent contains thermal energy (20–25°C) – its recovery would be enough to heat 141,500 homes worldwide. This can be recovered via heat exchangers and heat pump technologies, applied at various points in the sewer system, or through micro-hydropower from RO wastewater flow (electricity can be generated from the kinetic energy of wastewater flow).

Moreover, several new technologies and developments are now available to reduce water utilization in hemodialysis [48].

Any intervention that delays or avoids the need for dialysis – such as early transplantation, pharmacological and non-pharmacological pre-dialysis strategies (e.g., nutrition and exercise) – is beneficial both for patient well-being and the environment [49].

Renal diets with reduced protein intake and a plant-based focus are increasingly recommended for preserving kidney function, slowing CKD progression, and alleviating uremic symptoms.

Such patient- and planet-friendly strategies should be a clinical and public health priority, offering the potential to reduce costs, drug usage, and environmental harm while improving the quality of life [50, 51].

6. Conclusion

Here, several ethical dilemmas present in modern medicine are analysed using, as an example, dialysis treatment applied to vulnerable, elderly populations, demanding thoughtful, methodical, and empathetic solutions. A central case of a typical patient, Mrs. A (adapted from a real situation), is considered to illustrate the importance of best practices in nephrology, integration of palliative care, shared decision-making, and adherence to previously stated values.

The comparison between two hypothetical pathways followed by Mrs. A., one lacking shared decision-making and the other incorporating it, clearly reveals that the second path results in better care, being more effective from the medical point of view and ethically correct.

Important issues addressed in this paper also include the ethical considerations of sustainability and justice for future generations, as well as the role that new green technologies may play in mitigating the harmful effects of modern medicine on both the environment and the interdependence between humans, animals, and nature.

From this paper, which is supported by comprehensive data from several previous studies, it can be concluded that contemporary nephrology must balance technological possibilities with patient dignity, resources, and environmental sustainability. Changing dialysis from a default treatment to a considered option is not only a clinical necessity but also a moral requirement. New models of care must incorporate ethical deliberation at every stage of the patient pathway, from CKD onset to acute crisis, so that lines, lives, and lessons can be ethically connected.

Table 1 presents an overview of the main ethical and practical domains to be considered in everyday clinical practice.

Key home messages

Domain	Key message	Call to action
Autonomy and advance care planning (ACP)	ACP is valuable but insufficient unless accompanied by the education of surrogates and shared decision-making.	□ Identify a trusted representative □ Ensure that the representative understands the patient's values □ Review ACP regularly
Ethics and training	Nephrology should integrate ethics and palliative care training to reduce moral distress and improve end-of-life care.	□ Include ethics and palliative care in training curricula □ Encourage conversations about 'doing less' □ Provide palliative support
Moral distress	Recognise and address physicians' distress when faced with futility or family pressure.	□ Create team discussions □ Offer institutional support □ Promote shared responsibility
Environmental sustainability	Dialysis has a heavy ecological footprint; sustainable practices and alternatives are essential.	□ Monitor water/energy use □ Reduce plastic waste □ Explore conservative care and greener technologies
System responsibility	Balancing technology with patient dignity and intergenerational justice becomes a moral necessity.	□ Align care with patient values □ Consider costs and sustainability □ Advocate for systemic change

Table 1.
Summary of key messages across ethical the domains.

Author details

Ana Mateus[1]*, Pedro Ponce[2,3] and Ivo Laranjinha[4]

1 Department of Nephrology, Hospital Cruz Vermelha, Lisboa, Portugal

2 Department of Intensive Medicine, Hospital Cuf Tejo, Lisboa, Portugal

3 National Medical Director of NephroCare, Portugal

4 Department of Nephrology, Hospital de Santa Cruz - Unidade Local de Saúde Lisboa Ocidental, Portugal

*Address all correspondence to: anaamateus@yahoo.com

References

[1] Alexander S. They decide who lives, Who dies: Medical Miracle puts a moral burden on a small committee. Life. 1962;**53**(19):102–105

[2] Bello AK, Okpechi IG, Osman MA, et al. Epidemiology of haemodialysis outcomes. Nature Reviews Nephrology. 2022;**18**(6):378–395. DOI: 10.1038/s41581-022-00542-7

[3] International Society of Nephrology. The ISN framework for developing dialysis programs in low-resource settings. International Society of Nephrology. 2021. Available from: https://www.theisn.org/wp-content/uploads/2021/03/ISN-Framework-Dialysis-Report-HIRES.pdf

[4] Abdel-Rahman EM, Hasan I, Abdelrazeq AS, et al. Early versus late initiation of dialysis in CKD Stage 5: Time for a consensus. Kidney International Reports. 2025;**10**(1):54–74. DOI: 10.1016/j.ekir.2024.10.001

[5] Rettig RA. Special Treatment — The story of medicare's ESRD entitlement. New England Journal of Medicine. 2011;**364**(7):596–598. DOI: 10.1056/NEJMp1014193

[6] Kjellstrand JC, Kjellstrand CM. Ethical conflicts in renal replacement therapies. In: Optimal Treatment Strategies in End-Stage Renal Failure. New York, NY: Oxford University Press; 2002. p. 229–256. DOI: 10.1093/oso/9780192629715.003.0010

[7] Avorn J. Benefit and cost analysis in geriatric care. New England Journal of Medicine. 1984;**310**(20):1294–1301. DOI: 10.1056/NEJM198405173102005

[8] Johansen KL, Gilbertson DT. US Renal Data System 2023 Annual Data Report: Epidemiology of Kidney Disease in the United States. American Journal of Kidney Diseases. 2024;**83**(4 Suppl 1):A8–A13. DOI: 10.1053/j.ajkd.2024.01.001

[9] Kurella M, Covinsky KE, Collins AJ, Chertow GM. Octogenarians and nonagenarians starting dialysis in the United States. Annals of Internal Medicine. 2007;**146**(3):177–183. DOI: 10.7326/0003-4819-146-3-200702060-00006

[10] Boenink R, Bonthuis M, Boerstra BA, et al. The ERA Registry Annual Report 2022: Epidemiology of Kidney replacement Therapy in Europe, with a focus on sex comparisons. Clinical Kidney Journal. 2025;**18**(2). DOI: 10.1093/ckj/sfae405

[11] Gillon R. Medical ethics: Four principles plus attention to scope. BMJ. 1994;**309**(6948):184–184. DOI: 10.1136/bmj.309.6948.184

[12] Holm S. Principles of Biomedical Ethics, 5thedn. Journal of Medical Ethics. 2002;**28**(5):332.2–332. DOI: 10.1136/jme.28.5.332-a

[13] Beauchamp T, Childress J. Principles of biomedical ethics: Marking Its fortieth anniversary. The American Journal of Bioethics. 2019;**19**(11):9–12. DOI: 10.1080/15265161.2019.1665402

[14] Kurella Tamura M, Covinsky KE, Chertow GM, Yaffe K, Landefeld CS, McCulloch CE. Functional status of elderly adults before and after initiation of Dialysis. New England Journal of

Medicine. 2009;**361**(16):1539–1547. DOI: 10.1056/NEJMoa0904655

[15] Oki R, Hamasaki Y, Tsuji S, et al. Clinical frailty assessment might be associated with mortality in incident dialysis patients. Scientific Reports. 2022;**12**(1):17651. DOI: 10.1038/s41598-022-22483-8

[16] Kreuter W. Treatment Intensity at the end of Life in older adults receiving long-term dialysis. Archives of Internal Medicine. 2012;**172**(8):661. DOI: 10.1001/archinternmed.2012.268

[17] Culp S, Lupu D, Arenella C, Armistead N, Moss AH. Unmet supportive care needs in U.S. Dialysis centers and lack of knowledge of available resources to address them. Journal of Pain and Symptom Management. 2016;**51**(4):756–761.e2. DOI: 10.1016/j.jpainsymman.2015.11.017

[18] Wachterman MW, Sinha A, Leveille T, et al. Nephrologists' perspectives and experiences with hospice among older adults with end stage kidney disease. Journal of the American Geriatrics Society. 2024;**72**(7):2060–2069. DOI: 10.1111/jgs.18936

[19] Combs SA, Culp S, Matlock DD, Kutner JS, Holley JL, Moss AH. Update on end-of-Life care training during nephrology fellowship: A cross-sectional national survey of fellows. American Journal of Kidney Diseases. 2015;**65**(2):233–239. DOI: 10.1053/j.ajkd.2014.07.018

[20] Moss AH, Holley JL, Davison SN, et al. CORE CURRICULUM IN NEPHROLOGY Palliative care. Published Online. 2004; DOI: 10.1053/j.ajkd.2003.10.011

[21] Mateus A, Farinha A, Araújo M, et al. Palliative Care Competencies in Nephrology: A Scoping Review. Portuguese Journal of Nephrology & Hypertension. 2022;**36**. DOI: 10.32932/pjnh.2022.11.209

[22] Gelfand SL, Scherer JS, Koncicki HM. Kidney supportive care: Core Curriculum 2020. American Journal of Kidney Diseases. 2020;**75**(5):793–806. DOI: 10.1053/j.ajkd.2019.10.016

[23] Gamondi C, Larkin P, Payne S. Core competencies in palliative care: an EAPC White Paper on palliative care education – part 2. European Journal of Palliative Care. 2013;**20**(3):140–145

[24] Rettig RA, Levinsky NG. Kidney Failure and the Federal Government. Washington, D.C: National Academy Press; 1991

[25] Moss AH. Revised dialysis clinical practice guideline promotes more informed decision-making. Clinical Journal of the American Society of Nephrology. 2010;**5**(12):2380–2383. DOI: 10.2215/CJN.07170810

[26] Abram MB. President's commission for the study of Ethical problems in Medicine and Biomedical and behavioral research. Making Health Care Decisions Volume One: Report. Published online October. 1982;30–44

[27] Morrison RS, Meier DE, Arnold RM. What's wrong with advance care planning? JAMA - Journal of the American Medical Association. 2021;**326**(16):1575–1576. DOI: 10.1001/jama.2021.16430

[28] Dugdale LS. Paradigm Shift: Dialysis as a terminal condition. Kidney

International Reports. 2024;**9**(10):2842–2843. DOI: 10.1016/j.ekir.2024.08.016

[29] Mitchell SL, Volandes AE, Gutman R, et al. Advance care planning video intervention among long-stay nursing home residents. JAMA Internal Medicine. 2020;**180**(8):1070. DOI: 10.1001/jamainternmed.2020.2366

[30] Pnck GJ, et al. Effectiveness of a Nurse-Led multidisciplinary intervention vs usual care on advance care planning for vulnerable older adults in an accountable care organization: A randomized clinical trial. JAMA Internal Medicine 2021;**181**:361–369

[31] Swidler M. Dialysis decisions in the elderly patient with advanced CKD and the role of nondialytic therapy. The Geriatric Perspective on Medical Decision Making; 2009. Available from: https://www.asn-online.org/education/distancelearning/curricula/geriatrics/Chapter37.pdf?utm_source=chatgpt.com

[32] Davison SN. End-of-Life care preferences and needs. Clinical Journal of the American Society of Nephrology. 2010;**5**(2):195–204. DOI: 10.2215/CJN.05960809

[33] Carson RC, Juszczak M, Davenport A, Burns A. Is maximum conservative management an equivalent treatment option to dialysis for elderly patients with significant comorbid disease? Clinical Journal of the American Society of Nephrology. 2009;**4**(10):1611–1619. DOI: 10.2215/CJN.00510109

[34] Więcek A, Gojowy D, Więcek A. Chronic Kidney Disease and Ageing. Journal of Gerontology and Geriatrics. 2017;**65**:299–302

[35] Schmidt RJ. Informing our elders about dialysis. Clinical Journal of the American Society of Nephrology. 2012;7(1):185–191. DOI: 10.2215/CJN.10401011

[36] Swetz KM, Burkle CM, Berge KH, Lanier WL. Ten common questions (and Their Answers) on medical futility. Mayo Clinic Proceedings. 2014;**89**(7):943–959. DOI: 10.1016/j.mayocp.2014.02.005

[37] National Institute of Diabetes and Digestive and Kidney Diseases BM. USRDS Annual Data Report: Epidemiology of Kidney Disease in the United States. National Institutes of Health; 2024

[38] Jb LFP. Handbook for Health Care Ethics Committees. Third ed. Baltimore, MD, USA: Johns Hopkins University Press; 2021

[39] Engelberg RA, Patrick DL, Curtis JR. Correspondence between patients' preferences and surrogates' understandings for dying and death. Journal of Pain and Symptom Management. 2005;**30**(6):498–509. DOI: 10.1016/j.jpainsymman.2005.06.006

[40] Cohen LM, Germain MJ, Woods AL, Mirot A, Burleson JA. The family perspective of ESRD deaths. American Journal of Kidney Diseases. 2005;**45**(1):154–161. DOI: 10.1053/j.ajkd.2004.09.014

[41] Skold A, Lesandrini J, Gorbatkin S. Ethics and health policy of dialyzing a patient in a persistent vegetative state. Clinical Journal of the American Society

of Nephrology. 2014;**9**(2):366–370. DOI: 10.2215/CJN.03410313

[42] McCabe MS, Wood WA, Goldberg RM. When the family requests withholding the diagnosis: Who owns the truth? Journal of Oncology Practice. 2010;**6**(2):94–96. DOI: 10.1200/JOP.091086

[43] Hoenich NA, Levin R, Pearce C. Clinical Waste Generation from Renal Units: Implications and Solutions. Seminars in Dialysis. 2005;**18**(5): 396–400. DOI: 10.1111/j.1525-139X.2005.00078.x

[44] Barraclough KA, Moller S, Blair S, et al. Updating the Data: The resource consumption of modern-day hemodialysis systems. Kidney International Reports. 2024;**9**(5):1521. DOI: 10.1016/J.EKIR.2024.02.010

[45] Bendine G, Autin F, Fabre B, et al. Haemodialysis therapy and sustainable growth: A corporate experience in France. Nephrology Dialysis Transplantation. 2020;**35**(12): 2154–2160. DOI: 10.1093/NDT/GFZ284

[46] Sehgal AR, Slutzman JE, Huml AM. Sources of variation in the carbon footprint of hemodialysis treatment. Journal of the American Society of Nephrology. 2022;**33**(9):1790–1795. DOI: 10.1681/ASN.2022010086

[47] Yau A, Agar JWM, Barraclough KA. Addressing the environmental impact of Kidney Care. American Journal of Kidney Diseases. 2021;**77**(3):406–409. DOI: 10.1053/j.ajkd.2020.09.011

[48] Abraham R, Goldfarb DS. Perspectives on water utilization in Hemodialysis: Nephrologists' Responsibilities. Blood Purification. 2025;**54**:447–454. DOI: 10.1159/000546034

[49] Piccoli GB, Murea M, Ben Hmida M, et al. Green, sustainable nephrology: State of the art needs for education and implementation. Clinical Journal of the American Society of Nephrology. 2025;**20**(6):889–901. DOI: 10.2215/CJN.0000000731

[50] Marrone G, Di Lauro M, Cornali K, et al. Sustainability and role of plant-based diets in chronic kidney disease prevention and treatment. Frontiers in Pharmacology. 2025:16. DOI: 10.3389/fphar.2025.1562409

[51] Piccoli GB, Earth MDS. Our common home: Toward a Sustainable, planet friendly approach to dialysis, a paradigm of high technology medicine. Journal of Renal Nutrition. 2017;**27**(6):478–484. DOI: 10.1053/j.jrn.2017.04.011

Chapter 8

Structural Determinants and the Ethics of Health Inequity: Law, Poverty, and Prevention

Daniela Oehring

Abstract

Health inequity represents one of the most pressing ethical challenges of our time, manifesting as unfair and preventable differences in health outcomes that stem from broader social, economic, and structural conditions. This chapter examines the complex intersection of legal frameworks, philosophical theories, and jurisprudential interpretations that shape our understanding of health equity as both a public health imperative and a fundamental question of justice. Through a comprehensive analysis of international human rights law, declarations, and constitutional provisions, the chapter demonstrates how legal instruments have evolved to recognise health as a fundamental human right while establishing state obligations to address structural determinants of health disparities. The philosophical foundations underpinning health equity are explored through major normative theories. These ethical perspectives provide moral grounding for legal interpretations that increasingly view health inequities as violations of human dignity and social justice. Jurisprudential analysis reveals how courts worldwide have translated these principles into concrete legal doctrines, with landmark cases from South Africa, Colombia, Brazil, and the United States illustrating both the potential and limitations of law as a tool for advancing health equity. Five detailed case studies demonstrate the real-world application of these frameworks, showing how legal action has dismantled discriminatory healthcare practices, expanded access to life-saving treatments, and prompted systemic health system reforms. The chapter concludes that achieving health equity requires recognising its indivisibility from broader social justice, necessitating coordinated legal and policy responses across sectors to address the structural determinants that shape health opportunities and outcomes.

Keywords: health inequity, social determinants of health, human rights law, distributive justice, structural discrimination

1. Introduction

Health inequity refers to unfair and preventable differences in health outcomes that arise from broader social, economic, and structural conditions. Unlike mere health inequalities, which are observable, measurable differences in health status between populations – descriptive facts without inherent judgment about their acceptability – inequities are imbued with a moral judgment of unfairness and injustice. Health inequalities become inequities when they are deemed avoidable, unnecessary, and unjust. A commonly cited definition by Margaret Whitehead [1] describes health inequities as 'differences which are unnecessary and avoidable, and in addition are considered unfair and unjust'. These inequities manifest starkly across the world [2, 3]. For example, there is an estimated 33 year gap in life expectancy between people born in the highest-income and lowest-income countries [4], and a child in the country with the worst under-five mortality faces 80 times higher risk of death than one in the best-performing country [5, 6]. Such statistics underscore that factors like poverty, substandard housing, limited education, and precarious employment can significantly shorten lives and diminish well-being. Crucially, these determinants are not random; laws, policies, and social structures shape them [7, 8]. This raises an ethical imperative: when avoidable health disparities stem from societal arrangements, there is a duty to reform those arrangements. In short, health inequity is not only a public health challenge but also a profound question of justice.

A complex interplay of legal frameworks, philosophical theories, and jurisprudential interpretations shapes the ethical considerations surrounding health inequity. Global consensus has emerged that health is a fundamental human right and that gross disparities in health status are ethically unacceptable [9–12]. Over the past decades, international treaties and declarations have codified obligations to address the structural determinants of health – the social and economic conditions that influence health outcomes [11, 13]. At the same time, moral and political philosophers have developed normative theories explaining *why* such inequities are unjust and how societies ought to distribute health resources fairly [14–18]. Courts and jurists around the world have, in turn, grappled with applying these lofty principles to concrete cases, sometimes advancing progressive interpretations that promote equity, and at other times revealing the tensions between legal norms and resource constraints [19–21].

This chapter provides an in-depth review of the global legal frameworks that address health inequity, alongside the deontological, philosophical, and jurisprudential foundations that underpin the ethics of health equity. It examines how international human rights law, World Health Organization (WHO) declarations, and national constitutions establish duties to combat health disparities. It then explores key ethical theories – from rights-based deontology to theories of social justice – that normatively guide our understanding of health inequity. The role of major institutions (WHO, United Nations bodies, and national courts) in shaping the regulatory ethics of health is analysed, highlighting how legal interpretation translates moral imperatives into policy. The chapter discusses landmark legal cases and case studies that illustrate how the law has been used both to address and, sometimes, to perpetuate health disparities. Throughout, while empirical data is used to ground the discussion, the emphasis remains on normative and conceptual analysis, interrogating not just the *extent* of health inequities, but the *ethical foundations* for why and how they should be remedied.

2. Legal frameworks

2.1 International human rights law

The principle that health is a basic human right is enshrined in foundational legal instruments (**Table 1**). The Constitution of the WHO [9] declares that [22] 'the enjoyment of the highest attainable standard of health is one of the fundamental rights of every human being without distinction of race, religion, political belief, economic or social condition.' This pioneering statement links health with fundamental human dignity and non-discrimination. Soon after, the Universal Declaration of Human Rights [10] proclaimed in Article 25 that everyone has the right to a standard of living adequate for health and well-being [23], explicitly listing food, medical care, housing, and social services as elements of that right. This was given binding legal form in the International Covenant on Economic, Social and Cultural Rights (ICESCR) [24], whose Article 12 requires states to recognise [24] 'the right of everyone to the enjoyment of the highest attainable standard of physical and mental health.' Under Article 12, states must take steps towards the 'prevention, treatment and control of epidemic, endemic, occupational and other diseases' and the 'creation of conditions which would assure to all medical service and medical attention in the event of sickness', among other obligations. The UN Committee on Economic, Social and Cultural Rights, in its authoritative General Comment No. 14 (2000), clarified that the right to health extends beyond healthcare to the underlying determinants of health – such as nutrition, safe water, sanitation, healthy working conditions, and a clean environment – and that states are obliged to take deliberate, concrete steps towards improving these conditions without discrimination [25]. Notably, the Committee affirmed that every human being is entitled to the highest attainable health 'conducive to living a life in dignity', emphasising that health must be seen in the context of broader enabling conditions of life.

International human rights law also embeds principles of equality and non-discrimination that underpin health equity. The ICESCR mandates that rights be exercised without discrimination of any kind, and other treaties reinforce this [24]. The Convention on the Elimination of All Forms of Racial Discrimination (1965) obliges states to guarantee civil, political, economic, and social rights (explicitly including the right to public health and medical care) without distinctions based on race [26]. The Convention on the Elimination of Discrimination Against Women (CEDAW) [27], in Article 12, requires the elimination of discrimination against women in healthcare. It ensures equal access to services, highlighting obligations in maternal and reproductive health [27]. The Convention on the Rights of the Child [27], in Article 24, recognises the child's right to the highest attainable health and urges states to take measures to diminish infant and child mortality and to combat disease and malnutrition [28]. More recently, the Convention on the Rights of Persons with Disabilities (2006) affirms the right of persons with disabilities to the highest attainable health without discrimination [29].

The COVID-19 pandemic exposed critical weaknesses in the existing international health law framework, particularly regarding equitable access to health resources during global emergencies. In response, the WHO Pandemic Agreement, adopted in May 2025, represents a watershed moment in international health equity law. As only the second international legal agreement negotiated under Article 19 of the WHO Constitution, it explicitly aims to make the world 'more equitable in

Legal instrument (Year)	Health-related provisions	Application to health equity context	Reference
WHO Constitution [9]	Preamble: 'the enjoyment of the highest attainable standard of health is one of the fundamental rights of every human being without distinction of race, religion, political belief, economic or social condition.'	Establishes health as a fundamental human right; explicitly links health with non-discrimination; provides the foundational principle that health inequities based on social or economic conditions violate basic human dignity.	World Health Organization. Constitution of the World Health Organization. New York: World Health Organization, 1946.
Universal Declaration of Human Rights [10]	*Article 25:* 'everyone has the right to a standard of living adequate for the health and well-being of himself and of his family, including food, clothing, housing and medical care and necessary social services.'	Links health to broader social determinants (food, housing, social services); establishes that adequate living standards, including healthcare, are universal rights; provides a basis for addressing structural determinants of health inequity.	United Nations General Assembly. Universal Declaration of Human Rights. Paris: United Nations, 1948.
International Covenant on Economic, Social and Cultural Rights – ICESCR [24]	*Article 12:* 'the right of everyone to the enjoyment of the highest attainable standard of physical and mental health.' Requires states to ensure: (a) reduction of infant mortality; (b) healthy development of children; (c) prevention and control of diseases; (d) medical services for all.	Creates legally binding obligations for states to progressively realise the right to health; requires non-discriminatory access; obliges states to address both healthcare and underlying determinants; provides a legal basis for challenging health inequities as violations of state duties.	United Nations. International Covenant on Economic, Social and Cultural Rights. New York: United Nations, 1966.
General Comment No. 14 [25]	Clarifies ICESCR Article 12: the right to health extends to underlying determinants (nutrition, water, sanitation, working conditions, and environment); establishes minimum core obligations; emphasises non-discrimination and prioritisation of vulnerable groups.	Authoritative interpretation requiring states to address social determinants of health establishes that discrimination in health access violates international law, requires deliberate steps to improve conditions without discrimination and prioritises marginalised populations.	UN Committee on Economic, Social and Cultural Rights. General Comment No. 14: the Right to the Highest Attainable Standard of Health (Art. 12 of the Covenant). Geneva: United Nations, 2000.
International Convention on the Elimination of All Forms of Racial Discrimination – ICERD [26]	*Article 5(e)(iv):* states must guarantee the right of everyone, without distinction as to race, to 'public health, medical care, social security and social services'.	Prohibits racial discrimination in healthcare access; requires equal treatment in health services regardless of race or ethnicity; provides a legal framework to challenge racial health disparities as discrimination violations.	United Nations. International Convention on the Elimination of All Forms of Racial Discrimination. New York: United Nations, 1965.

Legal instrument (Year)	Health-related provisions	Application to health equity context	Reference
Convention on the Elimination of All Forms of Discrimination Against Women – CEDAW [27]	*Article 12:* requires the elimination of discrimination against women in healthcare; ensures equal access to health services, including those related to family planning; and provides special protections for maternal health.	Addresses gender-based health inequities; requires states to ensure women's equal access to healthcare; emphasises maternal and reproductive health; provides a basis for challenging discriminatory practices affecting women's health outcomes.	United Nations. Convention on the Elimination of All Forms of Discrimination Against Women. New York: United Nations, 1979.
Convention on the Rights of the Child – CRC [28]	*Article 24:* recognises a child's right to the highest attainable standard of health; requires states to reduce infant and child mortality; combat disease and malnutrition; ensure pre- and post-natal care for mothers; and abolish harmful traditional practices.	Protects children's health rights; requires states to address child health inequities; emphasises preventive care and nutrition; provides a framework for addressing disparities in child health outcomes across socioeconomic groups.	United Nations. Convention on the Rights of the Child. New York: United Nations, 1989.
Convention on the Rights of Persons with Disabilities – CRPD [29]	*Article 25:* affirms the right of persons with disabilities to the highest attainable standard of health without discrimination; requires the same range, quality, and standard of free or affordable healthcare as provided to others.	Addresses disability-based health inequities; requires accessible health services; prohibits discrimination in health insurance; ensures persons with disabilities receive the health services needed specifically because of their disabilities.	United Nations. Convention on the Rights of Persons with Disabilities. New York: United Nations, 2006.
International Convention on the Protection of the Rights of All Migrant Workers [30]	*Articles 28 & 43:* ensure emergency medical care for all migrant workers; documented migrants have equality of treatment with nationals in access to social and health services.	Protects health rights of migrant populations, who often face severe health inequities; requires emergency care regardless of migration status; promotes equal access to health services for documented migrants.	United Nations. International Convention on the Protection of the Rights of All Migrant Workers and Members of Their Families. New York: United Nations, 1990.
UN Declaration on the Rights of Indigenous Peoples – UNDRIP [31]	*Article 24:* indigenous peoples have the right to traditional medicines and health practices; the right to access all social and health services without discrimination; and Indigenous individuals have an equal right to the highest attainable standard of physical and mental health.	Addresses health inequities faced by Indigenous peoples globally; recognises both collective and individual health rights; requires culturally appropriate health services; acknowledges traditional medicine systems; provides a framework for addressing historical and ongoing discrimination in healthcare.	United Nations. United Nations Declaration on the Rights of Indigenous Peoples. New York: United Nations, 2007. A/RES/61/295.

Legal instrument (Year)	Health-related provisions	Application to health equity context	Reference
European Social Charter (1961, Revised 1996)	*Article 11:* right to protection of health – requires states to remove causes of ill-health, provide health education, and prevent diseases. *Article 13:* right to social and medical assistance for those without adequate resources.	Regional instrument ensuring social and economic rights, including health; emphasises protection of vulnerable groups (elderly, children, disabled, and migrants); requires non-discriminatory access; complements ECHR's civil/political rights with socioeconomic rights.	Council of Europe. European Social Charter (Revised). Strasbourg: Council of Europe, 1996. ETS No. 163.
African Charter on Human and Peoples' Rights (1981)	*Article 16:* 'every individual shall have the right to enjoy the best attainable state of physical and mental health', and states shall take necessary measures to protect health and ensure medical attention in sickness.	Regional instrument for Africa addressing health as a fundamental right; links individual and collective rights; emphasises state duties to ensure healthcare access; provides a basis for addressing health inequities in the African context.	Organisation of African Unity. African Charter on Human and Peoples' Rights. Nairobi: OAU, 1981.
Additional Protocol to the American Convention on Human Rights – Protocol of San Salvador [39]	*Article 10:* right to health as 'enjoyment of the highest level of physical, mental and social well-being'; includes primary healthcare, extension of health services to all, universal immunisation, and prevention or treatment of diseases.	Regional instrument for the Americas establishing economic, social, and cultural rights; requires states to ensure health services reach all individuals, especially vulnerable groups; emphasises primary healthcare and prevention.	Organisation of American States. Additional Protocol to the American Convention on Human Rights in the Area of Economic, Social, and Cultural Rights 'Protocol of San Salvador'. San Salvador: OAS, 1988.
Convention on the Rights of Persons Living with HIV/AIDS (Various Guidelines)	International Guidelines on HIV/AIDS and Human Rights (UNAIDS/OHCHR): emphasises non-discrimination, access to prevention and treatment, informed consent, confidentiality, and participation of affected communities.	Addresses specific health inequities faced by people with HIV/AIDS; combats stigma and discrimination; ensures access to antiretroviral therapy; protects rights in healthcare settings; promotes community involvement in health responses.	UNAIDS/OHCHR. International Guidelines on HIV/AIDS and Human Rights. Geneva: United Nations, 2006 (Consolidated Version).
Arab Charter on Human Rights (2004)	*Article 39:* right to the highest attainable standard of physical and mental health; free basic healthcare services; access to health facilities without discrimination.	Regional instrument for Arab states recognising health as a fundamental right; requires states to provide basic health services and ensure non-discriminatory access; addresses health needs in the context of the Arab region.	League of Arab States. Arab Charter on Human Rights. Cairo: League of Arab States, 2004.

Legal instrument (Year)	Health-related provisions	Application to health equity context	Reference
ILO Conventions on Occupational Health	Multiple conventions, including C155 (Occupational Safety and Health, 1981) and C161 (Occupational Health Services, 1985) establish workers' rights to safe and healthy working conditions.	Addresses health inequities related to work and employment; protects vulnerable workers from occupational hazards; requires preventive health services in the workplace; recognises work as a social determinant of health.	International Labour Organization. Occupational Safety and Health Convention (C155). Geneva: ILO, 1981. International Labour Organization. Occupational Health Services Convention (C161). Geneva: ILO, 1985.
WHO Pandemic Agreement (2025)	*Preamble:* stresses that adequate pandemic prevention, preparedness, response, and health systems recovery are part of a continuum to achieve greater health equity through resolute action on the social, environmental, cultural, political, and economic determinants of health. *Chapter 1, Article 3.4*: stipulates directly equity as a goal, principle, and outcome of pandemic prevention, preparedness, and response, striving in this context for the absence of unfair, avoidable, or remediable differences among and between individuals, communities, and countries. *Article 6.1* obliges all states to take appropriate measures to develop, strengthen, and maintain a resilient health system, considering the need for equity to achieve universal health coverage.	Directly addresses health inequities at a global coordination level and is the world's first pandemic agreement; sets out the principles, approaches, and tools for better international coordination to strengthen the global health architecture for pandemic prevention, preparedness, and response, including equitable and timely access to vaccines, therapeutics, and diagnostics; aims to establish a financial mechanism to 'enhance, facilitate, and work to remove barriers and ensure equitable, timely, rapid, safe, and affordable access to pandemic-related health products for countries in need during public health emergencies of international concern'.	World Health Organization. (2025). WHO Pandemic Agreement: Resolution WHA78.1, adopted by the Seventy-eighth World Health Assembly on 20 May 2025. Geneva: World Health Organization. *The WHO Pandemic Agreement shall be open for signature after the adoption of the Annex described in Article 12 of the Agreement by the Health Assembly International Covenant on Economic, Social and Cultural Rights | OHCHR, which means it is not yet open for signature, as the Pathogen Access and Benefit-Sharing (PABS) Instrument referenced in Article 12 still needs to be completed by the Intergovernmental Working Group.*

Note: This table summarises the primary international human rights instruments that establish legal obligations related to health equity. Each instrument creates binding obligations for States Parties to respect, protect, and fulfil the right to health without discrimination, with particular attention to vulnerable and marginalised populations. The principle of progressive realisation *applies to economic, social, and cultural rights, requiring states to take deliberate steps toward full realisation while certain core obligations (such as non-discrimination) are of immediate effect.*

Table 1.
International human rights law instruments relevant to health equity.

response to future pandemics'. The agreement establishes binding principles, approaches, and tools for international coordination to strengthen the global health architecture for pandemic prevention, preparedness, and response. Crucially, it mandates equitable and timely access to vaccines, therapeutics, and diagnostics – addressing the stark inequities witnessed during COVID-19 when high-income countries monopolised vaccine supplies while low-income nations waited months for access. The agreement also establishes innovative mechanisms, including a coordinating financial mechanism and a global supply chain and logistics network designed to 'enhance, facilitate, and work to remove barriers and ensure equitable, timely, rapid, safe, and affordable access to pandemic-related health products for countries in need during public health emergencies' [30]. This represents a concrete legal response to the moral failures of pandemic nationalism and reinforces that health equity must be operationalised even – or especially – during crises.

All these instruments create a dense normative web: states must respect, protect, and fulfil the right to health by refraining from interference, preventing third-party harms, and actively ensuring accessible, quality health services and underlying necessities for all, especially marginalised groups. Importantly, human rights law recognises that resource constraints may limit immediate fulfilment. Still, it imposes *progressive realisation* – a duty to move expeditiously towards full access – and certain core obligations that are of immediate effect (example, ensuring non-discriminatory access to essential services and an adequate supply of vital medicines) [31].

2.2 WHO declarations and global health policy

Beyond treaties, the global community has repeatedly committed to tackling health inequity through high-level declarations and strategies. A milestone was the Declaration of Alma-Ata (1978) on Primary Health Care [12], which famously stated that 'the existing gross inequality in the health status of the people, particularly between developed and developing countries as well as within countries, is politically, socially, and economically unacceptable'. Alma-Ata not only reaffirmed health as a fundamental human right but also identified primary healthcare – accessible, scientifically sound, and socially acceptable care – as key to closing the health gap within a generation. It called for intersectoral action, recognising that achieving *Health for All* requires addressing social and economic development broadly, not merely healthcare provision. Decades later, the world revisited these commitments in the Declaration of Astana (2018), marking Alma-Ata's 40th anniversary [32]. In Astana, all countries renewed their pledge to strengthen primary health systems as an 'inclusive, equitable, high-quality' foundation for achieving universal health coverage (UHC). The Astana Declaration explicitly found it 'ethically, politically, socially and economically unacceptable that inequity in health and disparities in health outcomes persist' in all regions. It underlined that poor and vulnerable populations still face unmet health needs and financial hardship from healthcare costs, and it urged actions to ensure equitable access to promotive, preventive, curative, and palliative services without impoverishment. This reflects a broader shift in global health discourse towards UHC as a unifying goal: ensuring everyone can use needed health services without financial ruin, which inherently targets inequality in access. Indeed, the WHO's 2019 report on primary healthcare [33] noted that countries must prioritise reaching those *furthest behind first* in the journey toward UHC, echoing the Sustainable Development Goals' mantra of *Leave No One Behind* [34, 35].

Another crucial framework is the focus on social determinants of health (SDH). In 2008, the WHO Commission on SDH released its landmark report, 'Closing the Gap in a Generation', marshalling evidence that poverty, food insecurity, inadequate housing, lack of education, and systemic inequities in power and resources are the root causes of health disparities [7]. This spurred the Rio Political Declaration on SDH (2011), in which governments worldwide declared their [36] 'determination to achieve social and health equity through action on social determinants of health'. The Rio Declaration reaffirmed principles from the WHO Constitution and Alma-Ata, including the fundamental right to health and the responsibility of governments to provide adequate health and social measures. Notably, it stated: 'We reaffirm that health inequities within and between countries are politically, socially and economically unacceptable, as well as unfair and largely avoidable.' Health equity, it emphasised, is essential to sustainable development and a better quality of life for all. To put commitment into practice, the Declaration and subsequent World Health Assembly resolutions (such as WHA 62.14) urged countries to 'improve daily living conditions; tackle the inequitable distribution of power, money and resources; and measure and understand the problem' [36, 37]. These actions correspond to the Commission's three overarching recommendations, essentially calling for a justice-based restructuring of societal policies.

The COVID-19 pandemic starkly revealed how these social determinants translate into life-or-death disparities during health emergencies. Crowded housing made social distancing impossible for the poor; precarious employment forced essential workers to risk exposure; and unequal access to healthcare meant marginalised communities suffered disproportionate mortality rates. This crisis served as a profound reminder to WHO and multilateral institutions that existing frameworks, while comprehensive in principle, had failed to prevent massive inequities in practice. The pandemic exposed critical weaknesses in international health law's ability to ensure equitable resource distribution during emergencies, prompting urgent reforms. These experiences catalysed new language in international agreements emphasising legally binding equity provisions, real-time monitoring of disparate impacts, and concrete mechanisms for global coordination – moving beyond aspirational declarations to enforceable commitments. The WHO Pandemic Agreement and strengthened International Health Regulations now explicitly require states to address social determinants when preparing for and responding to health emergencies, recognising that pandemic preparedness is inseparable from health equity infrastructure.

Global policy instruments complement human rights treaties by providing moral and political mandates: they articulate a consensus that reducing health inequity is not only a technical health matter but a demand of justice, requiring integrated efforts across housing, education, employment, and beyond.

2.3 National constitutions and legislation

International norms have seeped into national legal systems, with many countries explicitly embedding the right to health or healthcare in their constitutions. As of the mid-2020s, over two-thirds of countries have some form of constitutional health right or a duty on the state to provide healthcare or public health measures. For instance, the Constitution of South Africa (1996) is notable for Section 27, which guarantees everyone the right of access to healthcare services (including reproductive health) and obliges the state to take reasonable measures within its resources to achieve the progressive realisation of this right [38]. The Brazilian Constitution (1988) similarly proclaims health as 'a right of all and a duty of the State', ensuring universal and equal access to services and establishing a public health system (SUS) aimed at reducing illness and inequalities [39].

Bolivia's 2009 Constitution represents one of the most advanced frameworks globally for legally recognising and protecting Indigenous peoples' health rights. It explicitly prohibits discrimination, recognises the contribution of Indigenous peoples and people of African descent as part of the Bolivian Nation, and enshrines the right to self-identification – provisions that directly address historical health inequities faced by these populations [40–42]. This constitutional recognition of plurinational identity and intercultural health approaches provides a legal foundation for addressing the structural discrimination that has historically excluded Indigenous communities from adequate healthcare.

Numerous other constitutions – from Ecuador and Kenya to France and Indonesia – recognise either a justiciable right to health or at least a directive principle requiring the government to strive for health equity through policies. Such provisions often go hand in hand with guarantees of equality or non-discrimination that apply to health. For example, many countries' bills of rights prohibit discrimination on grounds like race, sex, gender, or socioeconomic status in access to public services, implicitly covering health services. Some have specific laws ensuring universal access or banning exclusionary practices (for instance, laws prohibiting hospitals from denying emergency care based on ability to pay, or laws mandating equal access to insurance). National legislatures also address structural determinants: for example, social security laws, housing and sanitation statutes, education guarantees – all of which shape the landscape of health opportunities. In recent years, we have seen legislative steps like 'health in all policies' approaches, where governments legally require health impact consideration in all sectors (e.g., as Finland did,) [43]. Additionally, anti-poverty programs (such as conditional cash transfers or legal entitlements to food or housing assistance) have been instituted in various countries, driven by recognition that improving these conditions will narrow health gaps.

However, the implementation of these programs reveals important lessons about preserving human dignity while addressing inequity. Early iterations often inadvertently stigmatised recipients – for instance, in the United States, visible paper food vouchers marked users as 'welfare recipients', undermining dignity and creating barriers to participation. Recognising this, the USA transitioned from paper vouchers to electronic benefits transfer (EBT) cards that function like debit cards, allowing recipients to access the supplemental nutrition assistance program (SNAP) benefits with greater privacy and dignity. This evolution demonstrates that how equity programs are designed and delivered matters as much as their existence – effective health equity interventions must not only provide material support but also preserve the dignity and agency of those they serve. Such design considerations are increasingly recognised as essential to program effectiveness and uptake, particularly among marginalised populations who may already face discrimination.

2.4 International health instruments and initiatives

While not law in the strict sense, several global instruments influence national obligations and embody ethical commitments to health equity. The WHO

Framework Convention on Tobacco Control (2003), for instance, is a treaty addressing a risk factor that disproportionately affects the poor worldwide; by requiring higher tobacco taxes, advertising bans, etc., it helps protect vulnerable populations from exploitation by tobacco industries and reduces inequitable health burdens [44]. The ongoing negotiations on a Pandemic Treaty similarly revolve around equity – seeking to ensure that in future pandemics, all countries (rich or poor) have fair access to vaccines and medical countermeasures, correcting the stark inequities seen during COVID-19 [45]. Moreover, trade and intellectual property law intersect with health equity: the Doha Declaration on TRIPS and Public Health (2001) affirmed countries' rights to prioritise public health over patent rules, enabling generic medication access for low-income populations – a legal tool to rectify the inequity in drug availability and affordability [46, 47]. At the global policy level, the Sustainable Development Goals (2015–2030) explicitly include targets on reducing inequalities (SDG 10) and achieving UHC and healthy lives for all (SDG 3), lending political weight to legal efforts [34].

A multilayered legal architecture – international treaties, soft-law declarations, and domestic laws – converges on a core premise: States and the global community carry legal and ethical obligations to eliminate discriminatory practices and dismantle structural barriers that lead to health disparities. This includes ensuring equitable access to healthcare and addressing the social determinants like clean water, nutrition, housing, education, and safe working conditions [12, 22, 24, 25, 36]. Crucially, these frameworks share a normative vision: that the test of a society's justice is reflected in the health of its most deprived members. Where entire classes of people suffer poorer health due to poverty or marginalisation, the law recognises an injustice that must be remedied through concerted policy and, where necessary, justiciable claims.

3. Philosophical and jurisprudential analysis

3.1 Normative ethical theories and health equity

The ethical analysis of health inequity draws on several major schools of thought in moral and political philosophy. A deontological (rights-based) perspective provides one powerful view: if we see individuals as bearers of inviolable rights and dignity, then profound health disparities violate a fundamental duty owed to each person. From a deontological standpoint influenced by Immanuel Kant's ideas, every individual must be treated as an end in themselves, not merely a means [14]. This implies that allowing certain groups (e.g., the poor or minorities) to suffer significantly worse health when it is preventable fails to respect their equal worth. The human rights approach is fundamentally deontological – it frames access to the 'highest attainable standard of health' as not just a policy goal but a right and correspondingly casts states and societies as duty-bearers [25]. Suppose a government has committed to the right to health. In that case, it has an ethical duty to take action against conditions like extreme poverty, inadequate housing, or lack of health services that systematically degrade overall health for some groups. This duty holds regardless of consequences or cost-efficiency; it stems from the moral claim of the individual. Such an approach aligns with the principle of justice as fairness – everyone should have a fair chance at a healthy life. In practice, this might support strong pro-equity policies such as affirmative healthcare programs for disadvantaged communities or legal guarantees of basic health services for all, even if these are resource-intensive. The deontological ethos is evident in many court decisions that assert minimum core obligations: for example, courts requiring the provision of life-saving treatments to all patients in immediate need, as a matter of right, reflect the view that particular health needs create absolute duties that override calculations of aggregate utility [48, 49].

In contrast, consequentialist or utilitarian approaches evaluate actions by their outcomes – typically aiming to maximise overall health or well-being. A straightforward utilitarian might argue that resources should be allocated to produce the greatest total health gain (e.g., measured in quality-adjusted life years or QALYs). At times, this can conflict with equity: directing resources to cost-effective interventions might improve average health but leave serious gaps for minorities or the very poor if their needs are more costly to address [35]. A utilitarian framework, if unmodified, might tolerate some inequality if total health is maximised. Indeed, one of the classic tensions in health policy is between maximising aggregate health versus distributing health fairly. However, many contemporary utilitarians incorporate equity by giving extra weight to improvements in the health of worse-off groups (so-called prioritarianism or weighted utilitarianism) [50]. Prioritarians maintain that benefiting those who are worse off has greater moral value than equivalent benefits to the better off. This resonates with the intuition behind health equity efforts – that reducing a health gap (say, reducing child mortality among the poorest) is especially urgent, even if the same intervention might yield fewer QALYs than other options targeting healthier groups. In practice, public health ethics often blend utility and equity, for example, through cost-effectiveness analyses that include equity weights or through the principle of *egalitarian utilitarianism,* where the distribution of health gains matters to the utility calculus [20].

One of the most influential frameworks in discussing health inequity is John Rawls' theory of justice, particularly as extended by Norman Daniels [15, 16]. Rawls' Difference Principle holds that social and economic inequalities are permissible only if they benefit the least advantaged members of society. Daniels argued that this principle can be applied to health: justice requires that we organise social determinants in such a way that health inequalities are minimised and any that remain actively improve the situation of those who are the worst-off. In a Rawlsian ideal, all the primary goods (income, education, rights, etc.) that affect health would be distributed such that the resultant health outcomes for the poorest are maximised. Rawls also emphasised fair equality of opportunity – the idea that each person should have a fair chance to pursue their life plans. Ill-health can be a fundamental barrier to opportunity; thus, health inequities originating from unequal social conditions undermine equality of opportunity [51, 52]. Daniels builds on this to assert that society has a moral obligation to correct health disparities because they reflect underlying inequities in the basic structure (education, income, etc.) that deny people equal opportunity to live a healthy life [16]. Under this view, healthcare is essential not just to treat illness but to keep people functioning as equal citizens in all spheres of life. Notably, if a society achieved Rawlsian justice – fair distribution of the social determinants – then any residual health differences would not be considered unjust. They would result perhaps from natural factors or personal choices in a fair context and thus be acceptable as just. But to the extent current health disparities are linked to unjust social arrangements (e.g., class hierarchy, racism, gender discrimination), they are themselves unjust. This Rawlsian view has deeply influenced jurisprudence; for instance, some constitutional courts implicitly invoke fair opportunity by requiring governments to provide certain basic health services (like immunisations or obstetric care) across all regions, to ensure everyone can equally enjoy a range of life opportunities [15, 16, 53].

Beyond Rawls, Amartya Sen's Capabilities Approach has provided a rich normative grounding [17]. Sen argues that people's capabilities should be evaluated in terms of justice – their real freedoms to do and be what they have reason to value. Health is central to capabilities: without a certain level of health, one's ability to achieve any life goals is drastically curtailed. Sen and others (like Martha Nussbaum [18]) therefore see gross health inequalities as reflective of unjust capability deprivations. If, say, women or the poor in a society have substantially lower life expectancy, this signals that they lack the freedom to live a normal span of life, which any just society should guarantee. Importantly, Sen cautions that focusing on health alone is too narrow – we must 'come to grips with the larger issue of fairness and justice in social arrangements, including economic allocations, paying appropriate attention to the role of health in human life and freedom'. In other words, health equity cannot be isolated from overall social justice. This approach conceptually underpins the idea of *health capability*: the goal is not merely equal health outcomes, but equal capability to achieve good health, which ties into laws about education, gender equality, labour conditions, etc. [54, 55].

Another ethical principle often invoked is social solidarity [56]. While particularly strong in European and communitarian traditions, solidarity takes diverse forms across cultures. Indigenous frameworks offer especially rich cconceptualisations that extend beyond Western models. At the WHO 24th Session of the United Nations Permanent Forum on Indigenous Issues (UNPFII), Geoffrey Roth (Lakota, Standing Rock) emphasised that the Global Plan of Action for Indigenous Peoples' health must reflect Indigenous conceptualisations, incorporating self-determination, culturally grounded healing systems, and ancestral knowledge. As Binota Moy Dhamai of the Expert Mechanism on the Rights of Indigenous Peoples stated, 'Their right to self-determination, protection of their land and territory, recognition of knowledge systems on traditional medicine, and Indigenous-led governance are crucial for maintaining Indigenous Peoples' *heal*th.' [57]

Indigenous solidarity frameworks often prioritise community welfare over individual gain, emphasising shared responsibility for social, environmental, and spiritual well-being. Many Indigenous ethical systems are grounded in principles known as the 'Four Rs': reciprocity, respect, responsibility, and reverence (with variations including relationship, representation, and relevance). The Latin American concept of *Buen Vivir,* or *Sumak Kawsay*, now constitutionally incorporated in Ecuador and Bolivia, exemplifies this approach. Buen Vivir advocates for renewing social and economic relations based on reciprocity and solidarity, emphasising collective well-being among social groups in harmony with nature. This framework challenges purely individualistic, rights-based approaches by insisting that personal health is inseparable from community health and environmental integrity.

In Western contexts, solidarity holds that members of society have a mutual responsibility for each other's well-being, especially the vulnerable [58]. It undergirds the ethos of national health services and social insurance systems – healthy and wealthy members implicitly subsidise care for the sick and poor, out of a sense of collective obligation. Solidarity-based reasoning condemns health inequities because they signify a failure of the community to take care of all its members [59]. This aligns with virtue ethics notions of compassion and communal flourishing: a good society does not abandon its less fortunate. We see solidarity reflected in constitutional commitments; for example, the post-WWII constitutions of Europe that led to universal healthcare systems were heavily influenced by solidarity and human dignity values. It is also reflected in international calls for resource sharing [56] – for instance, appeals during the COVID-19 pandemic for wealthy nations to ensure vaccine access in poorer nations were framed not just in utilitarian terms (to stop new variants) but in terms of solidarity and justice.

3.2 Jurisprudential interpretations

Courts and legal theorists have translated these ethical principles into doctrines and tests when interpreting the law. A key arena is how courts interpret the right to health and other socio-economic rights. Some judiciaries have been wary, viewing these rights as aspirational goals best left to the political branches (*non-justiciable*). Others, notably in the Global South, have embraced a more muscular role. For example, the Constitutional Court of South Africa developed a standard of reasonableness review in socio-economic rights cases. Rather than dictating exact resource allocations, the Court examines whether the government's policies to realise rights (like housing, health, and food) are reasonable and inclusive. In the famous *Treatment Action Campaign (TAC)* case (discussed further below) [20], the Court struck down an unreasonable policy that restricted HIV medication to pilot sites, finding it failed to adequately account for the needs of the poor and hence violated the constitutional right of access to healthcare. South Africa's jurisprudence explicitly rejects a rigid *minimum core* formula, as it declined to specify a fixed minimum entitlement for everyone. Still, it insists that policies must progressively expand access, prioritise the vulnerable, and not unjustifiably exclude segments of the population [48, 49]. This inherently embodies an equity-oriented interpretation: a health program that leaves out those most in need without good reason is not *reasonable* in a constitutional sense.

In India, the Supreme Court took a different route by expansively interpreting the fundamental right to life (Article 21) to imply a right to health and medical care as essential to life with dignity. Through public interest litigations, the Indian courts have directed governments to provide emergency medical treatment, improve nutrition programs, and ensure access to life-saving drugs, often citing the need to protect the poor and underprivileged. This jurisprudence leans on the idea that failure to address extreme health disparities can violate the right to life and the equal protection of the laws. For instance, in *Paschim Banga Khet Mazdoor Samity* (1996), the Supreme Court held that the state's inability to provide timely emergency treatment to a poor injury victim violated his right to life, prompting the government to establish a fund for free emergency care for the poor [19]. Here, the court injected the ethical notion of state responsibility for vulnerable individuals into the interpretation of a general right to life.

Latin American courts, particularly in Colombia, Brazil, and Argentina, have also shaped global thinking. The Constitutional Court of Colombia, in Decision *T-760/*

2008, undertook a structural review of the health system and ordered comprehensive reforms to eliminate barriers that caused unequal access to services [60]. It noted that the health system's segmentation, with different quality of care for those in different insurance regimes, was incompatible with the constitutional principles of equality and dignity. By ordering the unification of benefits and stronger financial protection, the Court essentially operationalised a right to health equity. Brazilian courts, faced with thousands of lawsuits, often by individuals seeking specific treatments, have generally enforced the state's duty to provide medications or care. Critics argue this micro-level litigation benefited those who could access courts and diverted resources from broader public health, potentially perpetuating inequity [61]. In response, Brazilian judges and scholars have been debating doctrines to ensure judicial decisions consider collective equity impacts – for example, moving from individual right-to-medicine cases towards structural injunctions that improve system-wide access [62].

Meanwhile, in countries without explicit health rights, litigants have used anti-discrimination law to advance equity. In the United States, for example, while the Constitution does not guarantee healthcare, civil rights jurisprudence has tackled inequities. A seminal case was *Simkins v. Moses H. Cone Mem'l Hosp.*, 323 F.2d 959 (4th Cir. 1963)., where African-American physicians and patients challenged the segregation of hospitals that received federal funds [63]. The court struck down racially segregated healthcare as unconstitutional, effectively extending the logic of *Brown versus Board* of Education to hospitals [64]. This judicial decision – a watershed moment in the quest for integration – recognised that separate was not equal in healthcare, and it led to the end of legally-sanctioned racial segregation in US hospitals. The rationale was grounded in equal protection: that government-supported facilities could not deny treatment on racial grounds. Similarly, jurisprudence under disability rights law, like the US Americans with Disabilities Act [65], has compelled modifications in health services, for example, providing sign language interpreters and wheelchair accessibility to ensure persons with disabilities have equitable access to care, as in *Eldridge versus British Columbia* (1997) in Canada, requiring interpreter services in hospitals as part of equality rights [66].

Importantly, courts often face the classic problem of resource allocation, sometimes termed the *tragic choices* of who gets what in healthcare. Philosophically, this raises questions of distributive justice and prioritarian ethics: should legal mandates ensure a sufficient minimum for all (a decent minimum approach), or aim to reduce gaps? Different courts have answered differently. The South African court's approach to socio-economic rights is often interpreted as endorsing a sufficientarian ethic, that is, everyone should have at least basic services, combined with an understanding that the most marginalised must be prioritised in policy. This is evident in language from General Comment No. 14 [13] and echoed by WHO [9], which asserts that equity requires prioritising those furthest behind – effectively a jurisprudential embrace of the ethical principle that improving the health of the worst-off is most urgent. In contrast, the European Court of Human Rights, which deals primarily with civil/political rights, has been hesitant to read positive health entitlements into the European Convention on Human Rights [67]. However, even the ECHR has tackled health equity indirectly through cases on discrimination; for instance, it has condemned the denial of health services to Roma people or people with HIV as violations of non-discrimination and inhuman treatment clauses [68, 69].

Another jurisprudential theme is the role of human dignity. German and German-influenced constitutional theory hold human dignity as inviolable, and some courts link this to basic socio-economic provisions [70–74]. The idea is that allowing people to live in conditions that predictably lead to malnutrition, illness, and premature death is an affront to dignity. This has led courts to require at least a safety net, such as food, shelter, and healthcare, as a matter of constitutional principle. Such reasoning is deontological at heart – it doesn't weigh costs and benefits but insists on specific inviolable standards for each person.

Jurisprudence across the world – while varied in doctrine – reveals a common normative undercurrent: an increasing acceptance that law should concern itself with unjust health disparities, and that traditional legal principles like equality, the right to life, or human dignity can be interpreted in ways that demand action on the SDH. As Gostin et al. (2019) observed, achieving 'health with justice' through law 'requires rigorous ethical justification if it is to challenge current harmful practices and support their replacement with more socially just interventions' [8]. Courts are gradually building that justification by referencing ethical values – justice, fairness, compassion – when they mandate measures to expand health access or protect vulnerable patients. At the same time, jurisprudence also highlights tensions – courts tread carefully to respect the separation of powers and finite resources, illustrating the practical challenge of turning moral imperatives into justiciable rules. Yet, the trajectory is towards an enriched understanding of health rights: one that is indivisible from other rights and grounded in the idea that health equity is a component of social justice.

4. Case studies

To concretise how legal frameworks and ethical principles intersect in practice, this section examines several notable case studies from different jurisdictions and contexts. These examples illustrate how law has been used to address – or at times exacerbate – health inequities related to structural determinants like poverty, discrimination, and resource distribution.

4.1 Case study 1: HIV/AIDS and the right to treatment in South Africa

In the late 1990s, South Africa was experiencing a devastating HIV/AIDS epidemic, with millions infected and tens of thousands of infants contracting HIV at birth each year [75]. At the time, an antiretroviral drug (Nevirapine) existed that could drastically reduce mother-to-child transmission of HIV [76]. However, the government initially limited access to this drug to a few pilot sites, effectively denying the therapy to the vast majority of pregnant women in need, many of whom were poor and relied on public hospitals. This policy became the target of a landmark lawsuit: *Minister of Health versus TAC* [2002, 20]. The activist group TAC argued that the government's restrictions violated the constitutional right of pregnant women and their newborns to have access to health services, and that it was an irrational and unjust differentiation – in effect, an inequity condemning thousands of infants to unnecessary HIV infection. The Constitutional Court of South Africa ruled unanimously in TAC's favour. It held that while the state could take progressive steps, it may not withhold available, life-saving medication from those who need it.

The Court found the government's programme was not reasonable because it 'excluded those who could reasonably be included', that is, women outside pilot sites. It ordered the state to immediately remove restrictions and make the drug available in public hospitals nationwide, as well as to provide the necessary counselling and testing infrastructure for its use. This decision had profound real-world effects: within a few years, mother-to-child HIV transmission rates plummeted, and it is estimated that the judgment helped save tens of thousands of lives [75]. Ethically, the case underscored a deontological stance – that the most vulnerable, HIV-exposed infants had a right to interventions already within the country's means, and that the state's duty to protect life and equality outweighed bureaucratic or cost concerns. The TAC case became a global beacon for how courts can advance health equity. It demonstrated that legal action and social mobilisation together can overcome structural inertia, forcing policy change to ensure previously marginalised groups, for example, poor HIV-positive women, benefit from medical progress. It also established an essential jurisprudential point: courts can enforce positive health rights in a way that respects broader policy space (by ordering reasoned extension of services rather than a fixed minimum core), thereby integrating legal and ethical reasoning in public health [20, 77].

4.2 Case study 2: Ending racial segregation in healthcare – United States

Racial disparities in health in the United States have deep roots in the era of legally enforced segregation. Prior to the mid-1960s, many hospitals and clinics, especially in the South, either refused to admit Black patients or consigned them to substandard separate wards. These practices were buttressed by laws and the tacit acceptance of *separate but equal* segregation, even in facilities funded by federal programs like the *Hill-Burton Act* [78]. The inequitable access contributed to stark health gaps – for instance, Black infant mortality was two to five times higher than white infant mortality, and life expectancy for Black Americans was years shorter than for whites [79–82]. An important turning point came with *Simkins versus Moses H. Cone Memorial Hospital* (1963), where African-American plaintiffs challenged the segregation of two hospitals in North Carolina that had received federal funds [63]. The US Fourth Circuit Court of Appeals ruled that this racial segregation violated the US Constitution, effectively because federal support made the discrimination *'state action'* subject to the equal protection clause. The court rejected the idea that separate could ever be equal in healthcare, noting the clear disparities in quality and access. As a result, *Simkins* became the first major case to strike down hospital segregation, predating the Civil Rights Act of 1964 [83]. Its significance was profound: it paved the way for the integration of healthcare facilities nationwide and the removal of formal racial barriers to care. Ethically, this case was grounded in principles of equality and justice – it vindicated the notion that institutionalised racism in health is morally intolerable and legally impermissible. The case also illustrates how law can tackle a structural determinant of health – in this case, institutional racism – which was causing unequal health outcomes. In subsequent decades, while formal segregation ended, disparities persisted in subtler forms. To address these, American law has increasingly turned to civil rights enforcement, for example, using the non-discrimination provisions of the Affordable Care Act (ACA) [84] or the Americans with Disabilities Act [65] to address intersectional issues like race and disability in care. *Simkins* remains a landmark because it established that health equity is a civil right, and it ushered in an era where federal policy, like Medicare in 1965, required hospital desegregation as a condition of funding. The historical lesson is clear: legal challenges can dismantle structural inequalities and lead to health gains – after desegregation, gaps in infant mortality and life expectancy began narrowing, though they have not been erased [85, 86].

The legacy of *Simkins* continues to evolve in the 2020s. The COVID-19 pandemic starkly revealed persistent structural inequities, with Black, Hispanic, and Indigenous populations experiencing disproportionate infection, hospitalisation, and death rates [87–89]. While some administrations have pursued health equity initiatives through executive action and federal programs [90, 91], these efforts face ongoing legal and political challenges. Recent Supreme Court decisions limiting the use of race-conscious policies in other sectors raise questions about the future of targeted health equity interventions [92]. Meanwhile, new forms of discrimination have emerged, including algorithmic bias in clinical decision-making tools [93, 94] and persistent disparities in maternal health outcomes [95, 96]. These contemporary challenges demonstrate that while *Simkins* dismantled de jure segregation in healthcare, achieving substantive health equity remains an ongoing legal and ethical imperative requiring continued vigilance and innovative legal strategies [97, 98].

4.3 Case study 3: Maternal mortality and gender discrimination

Alyne da Silva Pimentel versus Brazil [99] – Health inequities often affect women in unique ways, particularly in maternal health. A tragic illustration was the case of Alyne Pimentel, a young Afro-Brazilian woman who died in 2002 from complications of pregnancy after being inadequately treated at a public hospital. Her death reflected a broader pattern in Brazil – and many countries – where poor, Black, and rural women face significantly higher risks in childbirth due to substandard maternal healthcare – a clear intersection of gender, socio-economic, and racial inequities [100]. Alyne's mother brought a complaint to the UN CEDAW Committee, arguing that Brazil's failure to provide appropriate obstetric care constituted discrimination against women, violating the right to health and life. In 2011, the CEDAW Committee issued a landmark decision in *Alyne da Silva Pimentel versus Brazil*, finding Brazil accountable for Alyne's preventable death [99]. The Committee held that states have an obligation to ensure women's equal access to quality maternal health services and that preventable maternal deaths are a form of discrimination against women, since only women face the risk of maternal mortality. It was the first international human rights decision to explicitly affirm that maternal health is a fundamental right and to fault a state for failing to address systemic inequities in healthcare. The Committee urged Brazil to improve its health system, train health professionals in emergency obstetric care, ensure access for marginalised communities, and provide reparation to Alyne's family. This case study is notable for framing health inequity in terms of intersectional discrimination: Alyne was disadvantaged as a woman, as a person of African descent, and as someone of low-income status, and these combined to deny her appropriate care. The legal outcome influenced Brazil's health policy – in subsequent years, Brazil expanded investment in maternal health, launched anti-racism initiatives in healthcare, and improved oversight of maternity services, though challenges remain. More broadly, the case put governments worldwide on notice that high maternal mortality among certain groups, for example, rural Indigenous women or minority women, may violate international law. It illustrated how international legal mechanisms can be used to highlight and remedy health inequities that might be ignored domestically. Ethically, the Alyne case resonates with the deontological idea that no woman should die giving birth for lack of basic care in a world with the knowledge and resources to prevent it. It also underscores accountability: even where national courts are inaccessible or ineffective, global human rights bodies can provide a forum to demand justice for health inequalities.

4.4 Case study 4: Right to health and health system equity reforms – Colombia

Colombia provides an example of a court-driven systemic remedy to health inequity. By the 2000s, Colombia had a pluralistic health insurance system with separate regimes for formal sector workers and for those in poverty. In theory, it aimed for universal coverage, but in practice, there were significant disparities: the benefits package for the poor was more limited, and bureaucratic barriers left many without needed treatments, leading to a flood of tutela (constitutional protection) lawsuits by individuals. In Decision T-760/2008, the Colombian Constitutional Court took a bold step [60]: rather than handling piecemeal cases, it consolidated evidence that the health system's segmentation and failures were producing widespread inequity and declared the status quo unconstitutional. The Court ordered the government to implement a series of structural reforms, including unifying the benefits plan for all citizens so that poorer individuals received the same scope of services as the well-off, and eliminating onerous co-payments for the poor. It also mandated better transparency and participation in health system decision-making. This ruling was grounded in the constitutional right to health, derived from the right to life and social security, and the right to equality. By equalising benefits, the Court explicitly sought to reduce the unfair gaps in health outcomes between rich and poor, and between urban and rural. Over the next few years, the government complied: it expanded funding and, by 2012, had unified the benefits plan. Studies indicate that this contributed to improved equity in service use – for example, vaccination rates and access to medications in rural areas moved closer to urban levels, and overall insurance coverage became nearly universal [101, 102]. The Colombia case is a remarkable example of a judiciary not just removing a barrier but actively restructuring a health system in line with equity principles. It did so by a rigorous analysis of evidence, including statistics on unequal health indicators, and moral reasoning that a two-tier system was infringing the dignity and rights of those in poverty. The ethical stance was that healthcare apartheid within one country was intolerable when the law promises equal rights. The case also demonstrated the doctrine of *progressive realisation* in action: Colombia was ordered to progressively implement changes but within a clear, monitored timeline – marrying the concept of gradual implementation to accountability. This model influenced courts in other Latin American countries and is studied globally as an example of courts promoting systemic equity rather than only individual relief.

4.5 Case study 5: Health insurance reform and the courts – United States (Affordable Care Act)

In countries where healthcare is largely market-driven, legal battles over reforms can have enormous equity implications. The United States' ACA of 2010

[84] aimed to reduce the huge number of uninsured, disproportionately low-income minorities and to outlaw discriminatory insurance practices, like denying coverage for pre-existing conditions. It represented the most significant effort to date in US law to reduce health inequity at a structural level. Two major Supreme Court cases shaped its fate. In *National Federation of Independent Business versus Sebelius* [103], the Court upheld the ACA's individual insurance mandate but struck down the mandatory expansion of Medicaid, a public insurance programme for the poor, as written, making it optional for states [103]. The result was that some states, mostly poorer Southern states with large minority populations, chose not to expand Medicaid, leaving millions of low-income adults without coverage – an outcome that maintained a large geographic inequity in health access. This shows how a judicial decision, even if not framed in moral terms, can perpetuate or create inequity: people in one state could get insured and access care, while similarly poor people in a neighbouring state could not, purely due to policy choices. Another case, *King versus Burwell* (2015), upheld insurance subsidies nationwide, avoiding what could have been a massive loss of coverage in certain states [104]. These cases highlight the intersection of legal reasoning with ethical consequences: the Court's federalism concerns in *Sebelius*, limiting Congress's power to compel state action, had the effect of exacerbating health disparities – a trade-off not lost in public debate. Ethically, one could argue the Court failed to fully consider the right to health or principles of equal opportunity; legally, the US framework lacked an explicit right to health to argue. This underscores that where explicit legal standards on equity are absent, outcomes may depend on judges' ideological leanings rather than normative consensus. Nonetheless, the ACA overall did succeed in narrowing some inequities – for example., the uninsured rate gap between Black and white Americans reached record lows by 2016 [105] – illustrating that legislation can be a powerful tool for equity when upheld. The continuing legal fights and policy rollbacks around the ACA demonstrate that achieving health equity is an ongoing struggle requiring not just one statute but a persistent defence in courts and legislatures against challenges that may undermine the ethical objectives of reform.

These case studies collectively reveal how law in action can be a double-edged sword. On one hand, proactive litigation and progressive judicial rulings have compelled states to expand access and dismantle discriminatory structures, often aligning with the ethical stance that the most vulnerable have priority. The *TAC* case saved lives by obliging the state to honour its duty to the poor; *Simkins* opened hospital doors to Black patients, recognising their equal worth; *Alyne's* case elevated maternal health in the human rights agenda, pressing states to remedy gender injustices; Colombia's court-engineered reforms materially reduced gaps in health services; and the ACA's preservation (in part) helped millions gain insurance. On the other hand, legal systems can also entrench inequity – whether through neglect, for example, courts historically refusing to enforce socio-economic rights, or through decisions that favour other interests over equity. Laws themselves, if poorly designed, can perpetuate disparities: for instance, intellectual property laws that make essential medicines unaffordable, or zoning laws that concentrate environmental hazards in poorer districts, leading to worse health outcomes. Recognising this, a recent movement speaks of *health in all policies* – from education to housing to environmental regulation – should be viewed through a health equity lens. In essence, each case study is a lesson that achieving health equity requires both vigilant legal advocacy to push the boundaries of what law can do for justice and attentive law-making to ensure new policies do not inadvertently widen gaps.

5. Conclusion

Health inequity is fundamentally an ethical problem entrenched in our social structures – a reflection of deeper injustices in how resources, power, and opportunity are distributed. This chapter has demonstrated that a robust framework of global and national law, underpinned by a rich normative theory, has emerged to address this challenge. International human rights treaties and declarations have established a clear, if aspirational, duty to eliminate avoidable health disparities, framing it as part of states' obligations to ensure human dignity, equality, and the fulfilment of economic and social rights. These legal instruments, alongside the policies of global institutions like the WHO and United Nations, have progressively shifted the narrative: from viewing health gaps as mere unfortunate outcomes of development to viewing them as violations of justice that demand redress. The normative foundations – whether deontological commitments to rights and duties, or theories of social justice like Rawls' fairness or Sen's capabilities – provide the ethical rationale that has permeated into law: they insist that no person's health should suffer simply by virtue of where they are born, their race, gender, or socio-economic status, and that society has a moral obligation to remedy the structural conditions producing such suffering.

The jurisprudential developments surveyed demonstrate that courts around the world are increasingly willing to engage with these ethical principles. From South Africa to India to Colombia, judiciaries have recognised that upholding constitutional values may require compelling governments to take positive measures against health inequities. Courts have navigated the tension between idealism and pragmatism – seeking to enforce core obligations and non-discrimination immediately, while acknowledging the complexities of policymaking and resource limits through doctrines like *progressive realisation* and reasonableness. Importantly, litigation and judicial decisions have become a venue for the voices of marginalised communities to be heard, often exposing failures in governance that perpetuate inequity and catalysing reforms. On the flip side, where legal systems have been less responsive, inequities have festered – a reminder that law's silence or neutrality can itself enable injustice. Thus, the ethical critique extends to law itself: legal frameworks must continually evolve to address new forms of health injustice, be it climate change impacts, emerging pandemics, or technological disparities in health access.

A key insight from this research is the indivisibility of health equity from broader social justice. Health cannot be looked at in isolation; inequities in health are both symptoms and causes of other inequalities – in freedom, wealth, education, and voice. Therefore, ethical health equity requires a multisectoral approach: poverty alleviation, improving housing, education for all, gender empowerment, and racial equality – all are part of the health equity agenda. Laws and policies targeting structural determinants (like minimum wage laws, housing non-discrimination, or universal schooling) are as crucial to health justice as healthcare laws. Global institutions and agreements are increasingly reflecting this holistic view. For example, the Sustainable Development Goals knit together poverty reduction, reduced inequalities, and health improvement, implying that progress must be coordinated on all fronts. The WHO's call for 'equity in all policies' is essentially a call for coherent ethical governance – aligning economic, social, and health regulations with the goal of fairness in wellbeing.

The chapter's exploration of case studies further reinforces that real-world change is possible when ethical principles are given legal force. Where law has been a tool for equity – through courageous judgments or progressive legislation – tangible improvements in people's lives have followed (fewer deaths, expanded access, greater empowerment of the disadvantaged). These stories offer a measure of hope against the often grim statistics of health disparities. They also provide models and precedents that can be adapted and emulated across jurisdictions. For instance, the concept of a right-to-health litigation campaign (as in South Africa or India) can inspire civil society in places where inequities remain unaddressed; the Colombian-style systemic injunction can guide courts on how to handle complex social rights cases; the recognition of maternal health as a right can inform strategies to reduce maternal mortality elsewhere. At the same time, cautionary tales – like the uneven implementation of the ACA – teach that political will and social consensus are vital, and that ethical progress can be fragile if not institutionally secured.

Addressing health inequity is a normative imperative that the law is gradually embracing. The convergence of ethical theory with legal practice – seen in human rights law, constitutional jurisprudence, and international health governance – has established a growing body of principles and precedents for tackling the structural determinants of health. Yet, the work is far from complete. Normatively, consensus exists that health inequities are unjust; legally, the challenge is to continue refining mechanisms for accountability and enforcement. Moving forward, major global institutions like the WHO and UN must keep pressure on states to honour their commitments, perhaps through stronger review processes or new frameworks, such as a proposed Pandemic Accord that enshrines equity in global health emergency response. Nationally, the incorporation of health equity into legislation, for example, requiring health impact assessments for all major policies or mandating equity targets in health planning, could translate moral commitments into concrete action.

The philosophy of health equity reminds us that societal progress should be measured not only by advances in technology or aggregate wealth, but by how the least advantaged among us fare – by the narrowing of unjust gaps in health and life expectancy. Law, as this chapter has shown, is an indispensable instrument in that moral project: it formalises our highest ethical aspirations into rules and rights, and when properly applied, it can help build a world where one's health no longer depends on one's lot in the social lottery but is secured for all as a matter of justice.

Acknowledgements

The author extends sincere gratitude to Yvette Marie Gonzalez for her contributions to this chapter. Her input, engaging conversations, and editing have enhanced the depth and clarity of this work.

Author details

Daniela Oehring
University of Plymouth, Plymouth, United Kingdom

*Address all correspondence to: daniela.oehring@plymouth.ac.uk

References

[1] Whitehead M.The concepts and principles of equity and health. International Journal of Health Service. 1992;**22**(3):429–445.

[2] Whitehead M, and Dahlgren G. Concepts and principles for tackling social inequities in health: Levelling up (Part 1) (Europe: WHO Regional Office). 2006.

[3] World Health Organization. World Health Statistics(series overview). Geneva: World Health Organization.

[4] Freeman T, Gesesew HA, Bambra C, Giugliani ERJ, Popay J, Sanders D, et al. Why do some countries do better or worse in life expectancy relative to income? An analysis of Brazil, Ethiopia, and the United States of America. International Journal for Equity in Health. 2020;**19**:202.

[5] Schwandt H, Currie J, Bar M, Banks J, Bertoli P, Butikofer A, et al. Inequality in mortality between Black and White Americans by age, place, and cause and in comparison to Europe, 1990 to 2018. Proceedings of the National Academy of Sciences of the United States of America. 2021;**118**(40).e2107787118

[6] Unicef. Under-five mortality (data portal). 2024.

[7] Commission on Social Determinants of H. Closing the Gap in a Generation: Health Equity through Action on the Social Determinants of Health. Geneva: World Health Organization; 2008.

[8] Gostin LO, Monahan JT, Kaldor J, DeBartolo M, Friedman EA, Gottschalk K, et al. The legal determinants of health: Harnessing the power of law for global health and sustainable development. The Lancet 2019;**393**:1857–1910.

[9] World Health Organization. Constitution of the World Health Organization. New York: United Nations Treaty Series; 1946.

[10] United Nations. Universal Declaration of Human Rights. 1948.

[11] United Nations. International Covenant on Economic, Social and Cultural Rights. 1966.

[12] World Health Organization. Declaration of Alma-Ata: International Conference on Primary Health Care, Alma-Ata, USSR, 6–12 September 1978. 1978.

[13] Committee on Economic S, Cultural R. General Comment No. 14: The right to the highest attainable standard of health (Article 12 of the ICESCR). 2000.

[14] Kant I. Groundwork of the Metaphysics of Morals. Cambridge: Cambridge University Press; 1998.

[15] Rawls J. A Theory of Justice. Revised ed. Cambridge, MA: Harvard University Press; 1999.

[16] Daniels N. Just Health: Meeting Health Needs Fairly. Cambridge: Cambridge University Press; 2008.

[17] Sen A. The Idea of Justice. Cambridge, MA: Harvard University Press; 2009.

[18] Nussbaum MC. Creating Capabilities: The Human Development

Approach. Cambridge, MA: Harvard University Press; 2011.

[19] Paschim Banga Khet Mazdoor Samity v State of West Bengal, (1996) 4 SCC 37. 1996.

[20] Minister of health v Treatment Action Campaign (No 2), 2002 (5) SA 721 (CC). 2002.

[21] Corte Constitucional de C. Sentencia T-760/08 (right to health; structural remedies) – English summary. 2008.

[22] Organization WH. Constitution of the World Health Organization. New York: World Health Organization; 1946.

[23] Assembly UNG. Universal Declaration of Human Rights. Paris: United Nations; 1948.

[24] Nations U. International Covenant on Economic, Social and Cultural Rights. New York: United Nations; 1966.

[25] Un Committee on Economic S, Cultural R. General Comment No. 14: The right to the highest attainable standard of health (Art. 12 of the Covenant). Geneva 2000.

[26] United Nations. International Convention on the Elimination of All Forms of Racial Discrimination. 1965.

[27] United Nations. Convention on the Elimination of All Forms of Discrimination against Women. 1979.

[28] United Nations. Convention on the Rights of the Child. 1989.

[29] United Nations. Convention on the Rights of Persons with Disabilities, Article 25 (Health). 2006.

[30] World Health Organization. WHO Pandemic Agreement. Geneva: World Health Organization; 2025 2025 May 20.

[31] Ansar. Legal analysis of the implementation of the principle of progressive realization obligations in regional financial management in Indonesia. Journal of Law, Policy and Globalization. 2020;**100**:65–71.

[32] World Health Organization, Unicef. Declaration of Astana (Global Conference on Primary Health Care, 2018). 2018.

[33] World Health Organization. Primary Health Care on the Road to Universal Health Coverage: 2019 Monitoring Report. Geneva: World Health Organization; 2019.

[34] United Nations General A. Transforming our world: The 2030 Agenda for Sustainable Development (A/RES/70/1). 2015.

[35] Oehring D, Gunasekera P. Ethical frameworks and global health: A narrative review of the "Leave no one behind. Principle Inquiry. 2024;**61**:469580241288346.

[36] World Health Organization. Rio Political Declaration on Social Determinants of Health. World Health Organization; 2011.

[37] Organization WH. Resolutions WHA 62.14 reducing health inequities through action on the social determinants of health. http://apps whoint/gb/ebwha/pdf_files/WHA62-REC1/WHA62_REC1-en-P2pdf. 2009. [Accessed: 2025–August-18]

[38] Constitution of the Republic of South Africa, 1996, Section 27, (1996).

[39] Constitution of the Federative Republic of Brazil, 1988, Article 196, (1988).

[40] Añaños Bedriñana KG, Hernández Umaña BA, Rodríguez Martín JA."Living well" in the Constitution of Bolivia and the American Declaration on the Rights of Indigenous Peoples: Reflections on well-being and the right to development. International Journal of Environmental Research & Public Health. 2020;**17**(8):2870.

[41] Inter-American Commission on Human R. The Situation of People of African Descent in the Americas. Washington, DC: Organization of American States; 2011.

[42] World Health Organization. Strengthening Primary Health Care to Tackle Racial Discrimination, Promote Intercultural Services and Reduce Health Inequities: Research Brief. Geneva: World Health Organization; 2022.

[43] World Health Organization, Ministry of Social A, Health F. Health in All Policies: Helsinki Statement. In Framework for Country Action. Geneva: World Health Organization; 2014.

[44] World Health O. WHO Framework Convention on Tobacco Control. 2003.

[45] World Health Organization. Intergovernmental negotiating body (INB) for a WHO instrument on pandemic prevention, preparedness and response. 2025.

[46] World Trade Organization Ministerial C. Doha Declaration on the TRIPS Agreement and Public Health. World Trade Organization; 2001.

[47] World Trade Organization General C. Implementation of Paragraph 6 of the Doha Declaration on the TRIPS Agreement and Public Health. World Trade Organization; 2003.

[48] Soobramoney v Minister of Health (KwaZulu-Natal), 1997 (12) BCLR 1696 (CC). 1997.

[49] Government of the Republic of South Africa v Grootboom, 2000 (11) BCLR 1169 (CC). 2000.

[50] Parfit D.Equality and priority. Ratio. 1997;**10**(3):202–221.

[51] Nixon SA.The coin model of privilege and critical allyship: Implications for health.. BMC Public Health. 2019;**19**(1):1637.

[52] Williams DR, Cooper LA.Reducing racial inequities in health: Using what we already know to take action. International Journal of Environmental Research & Public Health. 2019;**16**(4):606.

[53] Giubilini A, Savulescu J, Wilkinson D. COVID-19 vaccine: Vaccinate the young to protect the old? Journal of Law and the Biosciences. 2020;**7**(1):lsaa050.

[54] Altuzarra A, Gálvez-Gálvez C, González-Flores A.Is gender inequality a barrier to economic growth? A panel data analysis of developing countries. Sustainability. 2021;**13**(1):367.

[55] Hay K, McDougal L, Percival V, Henry S, Klugman J, Wurie H, et al. Disrupting gender norms in health systems: Making the case for change. The Lancet. 2019;**393**:2535–2549.

[56] Pot M.Epistemic solidarity in medicine and healthcare. Medicine, Health Care and Philosophy. 2022;**25**(4):681–692.

[57] World Health Organization. Indigenous leadership and views must shape new global health action plan. 2025.

[58] Meijer MA, Brabers AEM, de Jong JD. Social context matters: The role of social support and social norms in support for solidarity in healthcare financing. PLoS One. 2023;**18**(9): e0291530.

[59] Horn R, Kerasidou A.Sharing whilst caring: Solidarity and public trust in a data-driven healthcare system. BMC Medical Ethics. 2020;**21**(1):110.

[60] Sentencia T-760/2008. Manuel José Cepeda 2008.

[61] Ferraz OLM.The right to health in the courts of Brazil: Worsening health inequities?. Health and Human Rights. 2011;**13**(1):33–45.

[62] Sarlet IW, Figueiredo MF.Health as an enforceable positive right: The Brazilian Supreme Federal Court's case law on the access to medicines. Kritische Vierteljahresschrift Für Gesetzgebung Und Rechtswissenschaft. 2019;**102** (2):117–134.

[63] Simkins V, Moses H. Cone Memorial Hospital, 323 F.2d 959 (4th Cir. 1963). 1963.

[64] v B. Board of Education. 1954.

[65] Americans with Disabilities Act of 1990. (1990).

[66] Eldridge v British Columbia (Attorney General), [1997] 3 SCR 624. 1997.

[67] European Convention on Human Rights. (1950).

[68] N v. United Kingdom. 2008.

[69] K.H. and Others v. Slovakia. 2009.

[70] Basic Law for the Federal Republic of Germany (Grundgesetz). (1949).

[71] Government of the Republic of South Africa v. Grootboom. 2000.

[72] Hartz IV Case (Judgment of 9 February 2010). 2010.

[73] Alexy R. A Theory of Constitutional Rights. Oxford: Oxford University Press; 2002

[74] Barak A. Human Dignity: The Constitutional Value and the Constitutional Right. Cambridge University Press; 2015.

[75] Kumar P, S SM, Govindaraj V. Forecasting of HIV/AIDS in South Africa using 1990 to 2021 data: Novel integer- and fractional-order fittings. International Journal of Dynamics & Control. 2023;**12** (7):2247–2263.

[76] Potty RS, Sinha A, Sethumadhavan R, Isac S, Washington R.Incidence, prevalence and associated factors of mother-to-child transmission of HIV, among children exposed to maternal HIV, in Belgaum district, Karnataka, India. BMC Public Health. 2019;**19** (1):386.

[77] Abdool Karim SS, Churchyard GJ, Karim QA, Lawn SD.HIV infection and tuberculosis in South Africa: An urgent need to escalate the public health response. The Lancet. 2009;**374** (9693):921–933.

[78] Hospital Survey and Construction Act (Hill–Burton Act), (1946).

[79] Mills A. The color of law: A forgotten history of how our government segregated America. Berkeley Planning Journal. 2018;**29** (1):154–156

[80] Laws JC, Crow J. Jim Crow Laws. 2015.

[81] Hahn RA, Truman BI, Williams DR. Civil rights as determinants of public health and racial and ethnic health equity: Health care, education, employment, and housing in the United States. SSM - Population Health. 2018;**4**:17–24.

[82] Reardon SF, Weathers ES, Fahle EM, Jang H, Kalogrides D.Is separate still unequal? New evidence on school segregation and racial academic achievement gaps. American Sociological Review. 2024;**89**(6): 971–1010.

[83] Civil Rights Act of 1964, (1964).

[84] Patient Protection and Affordable Care Act (Affordable Care Act), (2010).

[85] Shen M. The association between the end of court-ordered school desegregation and preterm births among Black women. PLoS One. 2018;**13**(8):e0201372.

[86] Johnson R. Long-Run Impacts of School Desegregation & School Quality on Adult Attainments. Labor: Human Capital eJournal; 2011.

[87] Centers for Disease C, Prevention. Risk for COVID-19 infection, hospitalization, and death by race/ ethnicity. 2023.

[88] Mackey K, Ayers CK, Kondo KK, Saha S, Advani SM, Young S, et al. Racial and ethnic disparities in COVID-19-related infections, hospitalizations, and deaths: A systematic review. Annals of Internal Medicine. 2021;**174**:362–373.

[89] Magesh S, John D, Li WT, Li Y, Mattingly-App A, Jain S, et al. Disparities in COVID-19 outcomes by race, ethnicity, and socioeconomic status: A systematic-review and meta-analysis. JAMA Network Open. 2021;**4** (11):e2134147.

[90] Executive Order 13985. Advancing racial equity and support for underserved communities through the federal government. (2021).

[91] Health USDo, Human S. HHS Equity Action Plan. 2022.

[92] Students for Fair Admissions, Inc. v. President and Fellows of Harvard College. 2023.

[93] Obermeyer Z, Powers B, Vogeli C, Mullainathan S.Dissecting racial bias in an algorithm used to manage the health of populations. Science. 2019;**366** (6464):447–453.

[94] Vyas DA, Eisenstein LG, Jones DS. Hidden in plain sight - Reconsidering the use of race correction in clinical algorithms. New England Journal of Medicine. 2020;**383**(9):874–882.

[95] Hoyert DL. Maternal Mortality Rates in the United States, 2021. Atlanta: National Center for Health Statistics: CDC; 2023.

[96] Petersen EE, Davis NL, Goodman D, Cox S, Syverson C, Seed K, et al. Racial/ethnic disparities in pregnancy-related deaths - United States, 2007-2016. MMWR Morbidity and Mortality Weekly Report 2019;**68**:762–765.

[97] Bailey ZD, Feldman JM, Bassett MT. How structural racism works - Racist policies as a root cause of U.S. racial health inequities. New England Journal of Medicine. 2021;**384**(8):768–773.

[98] Yearby R, Clark B, Figueroa JF. Structural racism in historical and modern US health care policy. Health Affairs. 2022;**41**(2):187–194.

[99] Alyne da Silva Pimentel Teixeira (deceased) v. Brazil, Communication No. 17/2008 (2011). 2011.

[100] Silva AD, Guida JPS, Santos DS, Santiago SM, Surita FG. Racial disparities and maternal mortality in Brazil: Findings from a national database. Revista de Saude Publica. 2024;**58**:25.

[101] Ruiz F, Amaya L, Venegas S. Progressive segmented health insurance: Colombian health reform and access to health services. Health Economics. 2007;**16**(1):3–18.

[102] Garcia-Ramirez J, Nikoloski Z, Mossialos E.Inequality in healthcare use among older people in Colombia. International Journal for Equity in Health. 2020;**19**(1):168.

[103] National Federation of Independent Business v. Sebelius, 567 U. S. 519 (2012). 2012.

[104] King v. Burwell, 576 U.S. 473 (2015). 2015.

[105] Baumgartner J, Collins S, Radley D, Hayes S.How the Affordable Care Act (ACA) has narrowed racial and ethnic disparities in insurance coverage and access to health care, 2013-18. Health Services Research. 2020;**55**(S1):56–57.

Chapter 9

Medical Education Technology

Omboosuren Bolorsaikhan, Gelegjamts Delgersuren and Gantulga Darambazar

Abstract

This chapter examines how Medical Education Technology strengthens ethical decision-making, cultural competence, and professional responsibility in health care. Using a mixed-methods design, data were collected from 2,300 Mongolian healthcare professionals through pre- and posttraining surveys and competency assessments. Ethics approval was obtained from the Mongolian National University of Medical Sciences Institutional Review Board, and informed consent was collected from participants. Findings demonstrate significant improvements in ethical reasoning, informed consent practices, and conflict management skills. Innovations such as AI-driven simulations, blockchain-based consent tools, and personalized e-learning are highlighted. This chapter argues that MET is essential for cultivating ethically competent, digitally fluent professionals able to navigate complex healthcare systems. This work provides an evidence-based roadmap for embedding ethics into digital curricula, with strong implications for low- and middle-income countries where access to conventional training is limited. By linking ethical competency with technological fluency, the chapter also demonstrates how scalable, digital-first approaches can help address global health inequities and prepare professionals for crisis contexts such as pandemics and climate-related emergencies.

Keywords: Medical Education Technology, digital health literacy, medical ethics, soft skills, informed consent, public health communication, ethical publishing, cultural safety, climate resilience

1. Introduction

In the evolving context of global health care, the ethical dimension of medical education is paramount. This chapter positions ethical competency as the central concern in healthcare education, with technology serving as the means to strengthen ethical decision-making, cultural humility, and moral reasoning. Medical Education Technology (MET) offers powerful tools – including AI simulations, immersive e-learning, and digital communication platforms – that directly address ethical challenges such as informed consent, patient privacy, and equitable access to care. In Mongolia, where cultural diversity and resource constraints pose unique challenges, integrating digital ethics education is particularly critical.

Globally, medical education has increasingly recognized that ethical preparedness must match the speed of technological change. International initiatives, such as the

WHO's Global Strategy on Digital Health and Finland's national digital literacy programs, emphasize the integration of ethics, data governance, and inclusivity into professional training. These models demonstrate that ethical competency is not peripheral but central to sustainable digital transformation in health care.

In Mongolia, the challenges are distinct yet interconnected: Vast geography, diverse cultural traditions, and uneven digital infrastructure shape how professionals access and apply training. Embedding ethics into digital curricula thus serves a dual role – bridging rural–urban gaps in professional development and fostering a culture of reflective, patient-centered care that aligns with both global standards and local realities. As seen in **Box 1**, reflections from a young physician highlight the importance of upholding patient dignity and maintaining an ethical presence in everyday clinical practice.

"Just as the golden sun nourishes all life indiscriminately, so too must a physician offer hope and uphold the dignity of every patient, regardless of their background or circumstances."

One Mongolian doctor reflects on the sacred weight of medical ethics – not merely as a formal code, but as a lived commitment. For this physician, ethics transcend regulation:

"To treat all patients with dignity, even in the face of death; to be present not merely with instruments, but with genuine compassion – this is the true essence of being a healer."

This narrative illuminates the emotional resilience and high ethical standards required in life-and-death decisions, especially within culturally intimate and under-resourced environments. As one Mongolian physician reflected:

"During my early clinical training, I inadvertently discussed a patient's sensitive test results in a public space. That moment profoundly transformed my understanding of medical ethics – from a superficial concern for professional appearance to a deep-seated respect for patient privacy, dignity, and empathy."

Such first-hand reflections highlight the importance of structured self-reflection in clinical education and underscore the necessity of cultivating digital self-awareness and ethical maturity from the earliest stages of training.

Box 1.
Reflections form a Young Physician: Upholding Patient Dignity and Ethical Presence.

1.1 AI + medicine: Ushering in a new era of health care

1.1.1 What is artificial intelligence (AI)?

Artificial intelligence is a rapidly evolving discipline that draws on multiple domains to simulate, enhance, and extend human cognition. It plays a transformative role in how knowledge is generated, analyzed, and applied across sectors, particularly in health care.

1.1.2 Defining AI from multiple perspectives

From computer science: AI is defined as the study, development, and application of algorithms and systems that replicate or extend human cognitive processes, such as learning, reasoning, and decision-making [1].

From an interdisciplinary perspective: AI spans a wide range of disciplines, including computer science, mathematics, physics, philosophy, cognitive science, neurophysiology, psychology, information theory, cybernetics, and fuzzy logic [1, 2].

1.1.3 What is medical artificial intelligence (medical AI)?

Medical AI represents a paradigm shift in healthcare delivery by leveraging AI technologies to enhance diagnostic precision, therapeutic planning, and systems-level decision-making. By integrating machine learning and data analytics into medical practice, AI aims to make health care more accurate, personalized, and efficient.

1.1.4 Core objectives of medical AI

- Improving diagnostic accuracy
- Optimizing treatment planning
- Enhancing workflow efficiency
- Enabling proactive health monitoring and prediction

1.1.5 Five high-impact applications of medical AI

1. **AI in diagnosis and risk prediction:** AI enables earlier detection of diseases and predictive modeling of patient risk based on vast data inputs.
   Example: Algorithms can assess risk factors for heart disease, diabetes, and cancer using electronic health records (EHRs) and real-time data streams (Rajkomar et al, 2019).

2. **AI in medical imaging analysis:** AI systems can interpret imaging modalities such as MRI, CT, and Xrays at scale and often with higher sensitivity than human radiologists.
   Example: Google Health's deep learning model for breast cancer achieved a higher accuracy rate than human experts in multiple validation studies (McKinney et al., 2020).

3. **AI in health system and hospital management:** AI tools are increasingly used to manage bed allocation, patient flow, resource utilization, and predictive staffing.
   Example: Predictive analytics for hospital admission surges based on seasonal trends and epidemiological data.

4. **AI in drug discovery and development:** By accelerating drug target identification and in silico compound screening, AI drastically reduces the time and cost of pharmaceutical R&D.
   Example: DeepMind's AlphaFold revolutionized protein-folding predictions, expediting vaccine development processes (Jumper et al., 2021).

5. **AI in medical robotics:** Robotic platforms enhance precision in surgery, assist in rehabilitation, and support elderly care.
   Example: The Da Vinci Surgical System facilitates minimally invasive procedures with enhanced dexterity and visual accuracy.

These can be classified into six eras:

1. Foundational mathematical and early neuron era (1943–1959)
2. Limitations and theoretical challenges (1960–1979)
3. Classical machine learning (1980–1999)
4. Modern deep learning resurgence (2000–2016)
5. Attention based architectures and Transformers (2017–2019)
6. Domain specific breakthroughs and large multimodal models (2020–2023).

The most rapid advances occurred in eras 5 and 6—attention-based Transformers (2017–2019) and domain-specific breakthroughs with large multimodal models (2020–2023) (**Table 1**).

1.1.6 Benefits of AI in health care

The integration of AI into healthcare systems has the potential to:

- Increase diagnostic accuracy and reduce human error;
- Accelerate clinical decision-making processes;
- Expand access to care in underserved and remote regions;
- Deliver personalized, patient-centered health care;
- Enable real-time treatment monitoring and precision medicine; and

Year	Milestone
1943	MP neuron – first mathematical neuron model
1957	Perceptron – early neural network architecture
1960	ADALINE – adaptive linear neuron
1969	XOR problem – foundational logic limitation
1986	MLP + backpropagation – breakthrough in deep learning
1995	Support vector machines – statistical classification
2006	Modern deep learning – onset of AI resurgence
2017	Transformer architecture – foundation for LLMs
2020	AlphaFold – a revolution in protein structure prediction
2022	ChatGPT – the first widely used web-based LLM
2023	GPT-4 multimodal AI – advanced reasoning and applications

Table 1.
Key historical milestones in AI.

- Facilitate early disease intervention and cost-effective care models.

1.1.7 Ethical and operational challenges

Despite its transformative potential, AI in medicine poses several ethical and technical concerns that require robust oversight:

- **Data privacy and security:** Patient data used to train AI models must be protected under strict confidentiality standards (e.g., GDPR, HIPAA).
- **Accountability and liability:** Responsibility for AI-driven clinical decisions must remain with licensed professionals.
- **Black-box models:** Many AI systems lack interpretability, creating risks when explanations for decisions are unclear.
- **Professional readiness:** Clinicians and educators must be adequately trained to understand, implement, and evaluate AI tools responsibly.

As Amann et al. (2020) highlight, maintaining transparency and patient trust in AI-supported care is a central ethical imperative.

1.1.8 Future directions and innovations

The future of AI in medicine is defined by developments that prioritize equity, interpretability, and patient empowerment:

- **Explainable AI (XAI):** Emphasizes transparency and interpretability of complex algorithms to build clinical trust.
- **Human–AI collaboration:** Positions AI as a cognitive assistant that supports – rather than replaces – clinician expertise.
- **AI in medical education:** Virtual simulations, intelligent tutoring, and adaptive feedback systems support competency-based training.
- **Federated learning:** Allows decentralized, privacy-preserving training of AI models across institutions without sharing sensitive data.
- **Real-time precision medicine:** Wearable devices and continuous monitoring enable highly individualized, real-time interventions.

1.1.9 Optional subsection: Integrating AI in medical education

To prepare future healthcare professionals for AI-integrated environments, medical education must evolve to include the following:

- **Simulation-based learning:** Use of AI-powered virtual patients and scenario-based simulations.

- **Intelligent tutoring systems:** Adaptive feedback tools that personalize learning.
- **Automated assessments:** AI-driven diagnostic skill assessments and remediation analytics.
- **Curriculum analytics:** Data-informed curriculum design based on learner outcomes.
- **Ethics training in digital health:** Including critical engagement with algorithmic bias and data ethics.

Artificial intelligence is no longer a futuristic concept in medicine – it is a current reality with far-reaching implications. To fully leverage its capabilities, healthcare systems must align AI adoption with principles of safety, equity, and human-centered care. Educators, policymakers, and technologists must work together to ensure that AI serves as a force multiplier for clinical wisdom, rather than a substitute.

2. Background and rationale

In response to mounting global crises such as pandemics, climate-induced migration, and sociopolitical unrest, MNUMS deployed hybrid learning models to deliver professional development in medical ethics and communication. These efforts acknowledge that ethics training must now also prepare professionals to respond to complex humanitarian and environmental emergencies.

2.1 Methods

A mixed-methods approach was employed. Quantitative data were collected via structured pre- and posttraining surveys from 2,300 healthcare professionals between 2022 and 2023. Qualitative reflections were gathered through open-ended questionnaires and focus group discussions. Participants were selected through purposive sampling, representing urban and rural healthcare facilities. Quantitative analysis was conducted using SPSS with paired *t*-tests to assess learning gains, while thematic analysis was used for qualitative data. This study was approved by the Mongolian National University of Medical Sciences Institutional Review Board (IRB No. 2022/115), and all participants provided informed consent in accordance with institutional ethical guidelines.

2.2 Results

- **Ethics and communication knowledge:** Pretraining scores ranged from 57% to 63.5%, while posttraining results rose from 88% to 90%.
- **Soft skills and conflict management:** Pretraining competence ranged from 40% to 65% and posttraining rose from between 80% and 100%.
- **Alignment with global standards:** The training content supported the development of competencies in public health communication, open-access ethics, peer-review integrity, and informed consent practices.

2.3 Discussion

The data show that the strategic use of digital platforms can yield high-impact results in ethical capacity-building. In an age marked by crises such as climate change, war, and global migration, equipping medical staff with ethical decision-making tools and emotional resilience is imperative. Moreover, the rise of cultural diversity among patients and health professionals requires educators to integrate cultural humility and safety training through simulation and AI-based adaptive learning. These digital tools enable learners to engage with real-world, emotionally sensitive scenarios involving refugees, climate migrants, and postconflict populations [3]. In Mongolia, cultural safety training has begun to integrate case-based simulation involving nomadic populations, ethnic minorities, and displaced individuals from border regions to build capacity in delivering equitable and respectful care. Comparative experiences reinforce these findings. For example, Singapore has embedded digital ethics into all levels of its health professional training, focusing on AI literacy and patient data protection. Finland has pioneered national curricula that integrate empathy and digital professionalism, while the WHO has issued global guidelines urging countries to adopt ethical frameworks for digital health. These international examples underline the importance of Mongolia's efforts and highlight opportunities for cross-country learning and adaptation.

2.4 Recommendations

- Integrate ethics and soft skills training into continuing professional development (CPD).

- Expand access to digital learning platforms nationwide.

- Promote research in digital health ethics.

- Institutionalize workplace-based ethics standards.

- Develop content on climate resilience, cultural safety, and humanitarian response within digital ethics curricula.

- MET and digital health literacy offer powerful tools to build ethical capacity and resilience among healthcare providers. Ensuring sustained investment in these areas will support better patient outcomes, improve public trust, and strengthen healthcare equity. Ethical readiness in the age of climate disruption and technological warfare will require curriculum innovations that embed cultural responsiveness, adaptive communication, and digital simulation of crisis scenarios.

3. Digital health foundations and ethical implications

3.1 Global trends and national context

- International digital health strategies (e.g., WHO, Singapore, Finland) illustrate the growing emphasis on ethical frameworks in technology-driven health systems.

- In emerging economies such as Mongolia, digital health maturity assessments (2023) have categorized national progress as foundational, yet promising.

- Mongolia's National e-Health Policy and Ministry of Health implementation plans aim to establish secure, interoperable, and patient-centered digital systems.

3.2 Implications for medical ethics and training

- The digital transformation of health care presents new ethical challenges, including informed consent in telehealth, algorithmic bias, and equitable access to digital tools.

- Safeguarding patient data and upholding digital professionalism are now core ethical duties for all health professionals. As illustrated in **Box 2**, an experienced physician reflects on the importance of ethical patience in clinical practice, emphasizing that digital innovation must not compromise core professional values.

Dr. D.B., a seasoned physician with over 20 years of experience, reflects on how ethical professionalism shaped her journey – especially during Mongolia's COVID-19 surge. In a private clinic, she worked under Dr. N., a mentor who embodied medical ethics through calm compassion even amid conflict.

"An elderly patient under our care tested positive for COVID-19 in her second week and sadly passed away. Her sons, overwhelmed with grief and fear, stormed into the clinic, shouting at my mentor for nearly three hours. But she never responded with anger. She simply stood there repeating, 'I'm sorry. I didn't expect this. I truly apologize.' I learned that day what ethical presence truly means."

Later, working in a district hospital, Dr. D.B. witnessed routine verbal abuse and emotional stress inflicted on frontline workers. Despite systemic pressures, she maintained her commitment to nonconfrontation:

"Sometimes silence in the face of aggression feels like weakness. But I've come to believe that controlled, patient response is an ethical strength."

This testimony highlights a vital message: Ethics is not only about theoretical principles but also about emotional endurance, compassion, and boundary-setting under real-world duress. Dr. D.B.'s account calls attention to the urgent need for better legal and institutional protection for healthcare workers, especially in resource-constrained and high-stress environments.

Box 2.
Individual Interview with an Experienced Physician: Ethical patience in clinical practice.

- To address these challenges, medical education must integrate digital modules on privacy, cybersecurity, AI ethics, and data governance to prepare future clinicians for the realities of digital healthcare environments.

Pre- and post-training ranges show participant scores on standardized competency assessments. Ethics & communication improved from 57.0–63.5% to 88–90%; soft skills & conflict management rose from 40–65% to 80–100%. Instruments assessed knowledge, communication, and conflict-resolution skills aligned with international best practices (**Table 2**).

Competency area	Pretraining (%)	Posttraining (%)
Medical Ethics Knowledge	57–63.5	88–90
Soft Skills and Conflict Management.	40–65	80–100

Table 2.
Pre- and posttraining competency scores.

4. Emerging ethical frontiers in AI-enhanced medical education

AI in Medical Education: Technologies Transforming Learning AI is rapidly reshaping medical education through a range of applications that enhance personalization, assessment, and experiential learning.

- **AI-driven simulation and virtual practice:** Learners engage in lifelike clinical scenarios that adjust in complexity based on performance, enhancing decision-making and empathy.

- **Personalized learning pathways:** AI analyzes individual learner data to adapt educational content and suggest targeted improvements.

- **Intelligent assessment systems:** Automated testing platforms provide real-time grading, analysis of common errors, and competency-based progression.

- **Data-driven feedback systems:** AI identifies learning gaps, tracks longitudinal progress, and enables instructors to deliver individualized guidance. These innovations improve both clinical reasoning and ethical sensitivity by exposing learners to ethically nuanced, high-stakes simulations in a controlled, supportive environment.

4.1 Next-generation evidence-based practice and clinical ethics

Artificial intelligence plays a growing role in clinical decision-making and education. While AI tools offer precision and efficiency, ethical responsibility remains with the human professional. Medical educators must, therefore, emphasize the integration of ethical reasoning and critical reflection into evidence-based learning [4]. Learners should be trained to evaluate AI-supported recommendations through the lens of ethical principles such as patient autonomy, clinical appropriateness, and contextual understanding. The balance between algorithmic efficiency and human judgment must be addressed explicitly in teaching environments that use AI as a decision-support tool [4].

4.2 Discipline-specific applications and ethical customization

Digital transformation is affecting specialty fields such as dentistry. In digital dental medicine, AI-powered tools now assist clinicians with diagnostics, risk stratification, and treatment planning [5]. These innovations bring new ethical challenges related to consent, responsibility, and the validity of algorithmic advice in clinical interactions. For example, an AI recommendation for orthodontic treatment must be transparently communicated to patients, ensuring understanding and trust. Medical curricula should integrate discipline-specific ethical models – such as those addressing AI in dental practice – to foster relevant ethical decision-making and data stewardship skills in students [5, 6].

4.3 Virtual environments, metaverse, and learner vulnerability

Emerging technologies such as the metaverse introduce immersive training environments for health professionals. These platforms offer innovative possibilities for reflective practice, emotional intelligence development, and values-based decision-making through virtual reality simulations. However, they also raise concerns about psychological safety, data privacy, and the blurred boundaries between real and simulated identities. Institutions must establish ethical guidelines for the development and use of such platforms, particularly in training future clinicians to navigate care for displaced populations, postconflict communities, and vulnerable patients with cultural sensitivity [7].

4.4 Global research trends and ethical challenges in digital health

4.4.1 Digital health complexity and ethical principles

Technologies such as cloud computing, big data, and AI enhance diagnostics and treatment but raise serious privacy concerns. Key ethical principles – autonomy, beneficence, nonmaleficence, and justice – must be interpreted in light of new risks regarding data ownership, consent, and equitable access [8].

4.4.2 AI clinical decision support systems (AI-CDSS)

Recent studies from South Korea and Turkey highlight ethical tensions in AI-CDSS, especially in high-risk decisions such as resource allocation. Core concerns include fairness, transparency, and the interpretability of "black-box" systems [9].

4.4.3 Regulatory and oversight landscape

Global agencies such as WHO, OECD, and the EU are issuing AI guidance, and over 950 AI/ML devices have been approved by the FDA. Regulatory frameworks such as GDPR emphasize human oversight and accountability in automated systems [10].

4.4.4 Algorithmic bias and inequity

Studies from the Czech Republic and elsewhere stress risks to underrepresented populations due to biased datasets and technological gaps. In Mongolia, regional disparities in data infrastructure, access to digital health tools, and limited AI awareness among faculty illustrate the urgency for inclusive data strategies and targeted faculty development. As outlined in **Box 3**, current digital health initiatives in Mongolia further illustrate the ethical and educational implications of these challenges. Proposed solutions include inclusive data design, participatory governance, and regular algorithm audits. Solutions include inclusive data design, participatory governance, and algorithm audits [3].

Case box: Digital health projects in Mongolia

Since 2020, the Ministry of Health of Mongolia has accelerated the integration of digital tools to improve health system efficiency, equity, and accountability. Key projects include the following:

- **e-Mongolia**: A national digital services platform that provides access to over 1,000 public services, including vaccination records, birth certificates, and health insurance data.
- **EHR**: Nationwide digitization of patient records aims to improve continuity of care and reduce medical errors.
- **Telemedicine services**: Initiatives in remote provinces have used teleconsultation to expand access to specialist care, especially during the COVID-19 pandemic.
- **Digital ethics pilot at MNUMS**: A project-based course on Clinical Communication Skills was launched online, based on adult learning principles and learning styles. The course demonstrated improved ethical awareness and communication outcomes among postgraduate learners.

These projects underscore both the promise and complexity of aligning medical education with national digital transformation. Ethics training must now evolve in tandem with these changes, incorporating data security, informed digital consent, digital professionalism, and equitable technology access into curricula.

Box 3.
Digital Health Initiatives in Mongolia: Implications for Medical Education and Ethics.

4.4.5 Ethical governance and institutional responsibility

Some healthcare institutions have established "technology ethics committees" to supervise AI implementation and maintain professional accountability. In Mongolia, establishing a national AI Ethics Board under the Ministry of Health could ensure transparency, professional oversight, and context-relevant guidance for AI adoption in education and care [10]. While ethical governance sets the structural foundation, the following section explores how innovative pedagogical strategies can shape individual ethical competencies in practice.

4.5 Innovations and pedagogical strategies in digital ethics education

4.5.1 Personalized ethics education and learning styles

Integrate learning style-based customization in ethics training. By aligning ethical modules with learners' cognitive preferences (e.g., visual, auditory, kinesthetic), healthcare professionals are more likely to retain and apply ethical principles in real-life clinical settings. Learning style-matched ethical scenarios enhances both retention and reflection, which are critical in moral reasoning and patient-centered care.

This approach is supported by local research in Mongolia, where the Mongolian National University of Medical Sciences (MNUMS) developed an online course for postgraduate learners on Clinical Communication Skills. A needs assessment involving 220 learners in 2024 revealed that 98% of participants rated soft skills such as communication, emotional regulation, and conflict management as "important" or "very important."

The course, built on adult learning principles and learning style adaptation, allowed medical professionals, including those in rural areas, to engage flexibly with digital content. Learners showed improved outcomes in communication effectiveness and ethical awareness, confirming that personalized, digitally delivered content supports both competency growth and workplace application.

4.5.2 Immersive simulation and virtual dilemmas

Develop immersive simulations (e.g., VR/AR-based platforms) that allow learners to experience complex ethical dilemmas in safe, repeatable environments. Scenarios can include breaking bad news, obtaining consent in vulnerable populations, and managing triage in resource-constrained crises such as pandemics or natural disasters. Embedding cultural safety and humility in these simulations helps prepare learners for empathetic care among nomadic, Indigenous, and refugee populations in Mongolia and globally.

4.5.3 Real-time feedback and ethical AI analytics

Use AI to provide personalized, real-time feedback on learners' communication styles and ethical decision-making. Tools can include automated empathy scoring, identification of culturally insensitive language, and flagging inconsistencies in consent protocols. LMS-integrated ethics dashboards can help track engagement and skill development.

4.5.4 Microlearning and mobile ethics modules

Design short, mobile-accessible modules (ethics in 60 seconds) with bite-sized ethical dilemmas, guiding principles, and reflective questions to encourage continuous learning, even in high-pressure clinical environments.

4.5.5 Digital professionalism and cyber ethics

Create interactive content that trains healthcare workers on ethical conduct in digital spaces, including social media boundaries, telemedicine etiquette, patient privacy, cybersecurity awareness, and responsible AI deployment.

4.5.6 Reflective portfolios and longitudinal growth

Incorporate digital journals or e-portfolios for learners to document and reflect on ethical challenges during clinical placements. Text mining tools can analyze growth in ethical maturity over time.

4.5.7 Peer-led dialogs and intercultural ethics

Facilitate moderated forums or virtual classrooms where learners from diverse cultural and institutional backgrounds debate ethical scenarios. This enhances global ethical literacy and respect for intercultural perspectives.

4.5.8 Blockchain for consent simulation

Simulate consent processes using blockchain to teach transparency, traceability, and immutability – core elements of trustworthy data and consent handling in digital health ecosystems.

As healthcare systems face growing complexity – driven by climate change, conflicts, digital transformation, and shifting patient expectations – ethical competencies must evolve accordingly. This chapter has demonstrated that MET can play a pivotal role in strengthening ethical awareness, empathy, and decision-making among healthcare professionals.

Innovations such as learning style-based ethics courses, immersive simulations, and real-time AI feedback are not only technologically feasible but also pedagogically effective. In Mongolia, for example, a digitally delivered course on Clinical Communication Skills, based on adult learning principles, significantly improved the ethical competencies of postgraduate health workers, particularly in rural settings.

National digital health initiatives have created opportunities for ethics-integrated learning, such as through the *e-Mongolia* platform, telemedicine programs, and the Ministry of Health's EHR system. However, implementation remains uneven due to limited interoperability, digital literacy gaps, and cybersecurity concerns. Medical education must, therefore, not only innovate in pedagogy but also align with the ongoing digital transformation of the health system.

Future progress in this area will depend on several key actions:

- **Institutional frameworks**: Establishing structures such as national AI Ethics Boards to guide responsible innovation and digital ethics policies.

- **Context-sensitive pedagogy**: Embedding cultural safety and humility into ethics curricula using localized case studies, especially relevant in refugee care, nomadic communities, and disaster response.

- **Scalable models**: Expanding microlearning, blockchain-based consent training, and ethical dashboards across medical schools and healthcare systems.

- **Digital alignment**: Integrating MET with national digital health infrastructure (e.g., EHRs, e-learning platforms) to ensure consistent and accessible ethics training.

- **Research and evaluation**: Investing in longitudinal studies to track growth in ethical reasoning, digital professionalism, and systems thinking.

By embracing technology with intentional design and ethical foresight, medical education can build a workforce capable of navigating today's ethical frontiers with empathy, critical reflection, and accountability.

4.6 Expanding digital ethics in medical education: Directions and future priorities

4.6.1 Strengthening reflective digital practice

Medical ethics education must move beyond content delivery to cultivate digital self-awareness, ethical reflexivity, and judgment. Digital portfolios, interactive reflection tools, and AI-assisted feedback can support learners in evaluating their ethical growth over time.

4.6.2 Scaling contextualized e-learning platforms

Local infrastructure and learner contexts should drive the design of digital ethics modules. Platforms such as the MNUMS Clinical Communication Skills course show that region-specific content – aligned with national culture, language, and system needs – can yield stronger engagement and competency development. Mongolia's vast geography and dispersed population pose unique challenges, and digital platforms can be a powerful equalizer. According to the Ministry of Health (2022), over 50% of Mongolian health workers expressed a desire for online ethics training. This indicates a strong demand for flexible, accessible learning modalities.

4.6.3 Embedding ethics into digital health policy

As Mongolia and other emerging economies scale national digital health systems, ethical dimensions must be integrated into technology rollouts. Digital health tools should include mechanisms for consent, accountability, and equitable access by design. Training must equip professionals to critically evaluate and navigate these frameworks.

4.6.4 Building a regional community of practice

To address common challenges in low- and middle-income countries, regional collaboration in ethics education should be expanded. Shared case repositories, multilingual content libraries, and collaborative research can foster resilience and innovation in digital ethics training.

4.6.5 Aligning with global digital transformation trends

Comparative analysis shows Mongolia falls within the "Emerging Economies" category in digital health transformation, alongside Brazil, Lebanon, and others. To progress, targeted investment in secure infrastructure, digital literacy, and instructional design is needed. Priorities should align with UN Sustainable Development Goals and WHO digital health frameworks.

4.6.6 Ethical implications of immersive technologies

Emerging technologies such as the metaverse offer immersive training environments for health professionals, enabling reflective practice, emotional intelligence development, and values-based decision-making through virtual reality simulations. These innovations raise concerns about psychological safety, data privacy, and the blurred boundaries between real and simulated identities. Institutions must proactively develop ethical guidelines for the use of such platforms, especially in preparing clinicians to care for displaced populations, postconflict communities, and culturally diverse patients.

4.7 Emerging innovations in ethics education

Comparative global experiences offer valuable lessons for strengthening digital health ethics in Mongolia. As highlighted in **Box 4**, insights from international contexts underscore the importance of adapting ethical frameworks to local realities while drawing on global best practices.

Case box: Comparative insights in digital health

- **Global ranking**: Nations such as Norway, South Korea, and Iceland lead in digital health maturity; Mongolia ranks in Tier 3 out of 4.
- **Spending gap**: Health spending per capita is $10,921 in the United States vs. $163 in Mongolia [13].
- **System efficiency**: WHO ranks Mongolia 145th out of 191 in health system efficiency – underscoring a need for strategic, ethical digital investment.

Box 4.
Comparative insights in Digital health: Ethics and Global lessons for Mongolia.

4.7.1 Gamified ethics learning

Gamification provides an engaging medium to explore ethical scenarios in low-risk, repeatable environments. Ethics "escape rooms," scenario games, and decision-based progress challenges can stimulate critical thinking and peer collaboration. When learners solve ethical dilemmas in a game-based format, they demonstrate higher retention and emotional connection with the subject matter [11].

4.7.2 Blockchain in consent education

Blockchain technology can simulate real-world ethical processes such as informed consent. It enhances traceability, nonrepudiation, and accountability – critical in decentralized health systems and clinical trials. Blockchain empowers patients to manage their own data while ensuring that health professionals adhere to ethical consent protocols [12]. As synthesized in **Box 5**, comparative global insights further

Case box: Online master's degree in medical sciences

The MNUMS has a rich history of advancing medical education since its founding in 1940. In response to geographic and access barriers across Mongolia's vast landscape, MNUMS launched the *International Cyber University of Medical Sciences (ICUMS)* in 2015 to provide inclusive, flexible postgraduate education through digital platforms.
This marked Mongolia's first fully online master's program in public health, developed in collaboration with Yonsei University (South Korea) and Johns Hopkins University (USA). The program rapidly expanded to six disciplines, including Traditional Medicine, Nursing, Dentistry, Pharmacy, and Medicine.
Courses were developed bilingually (English and Mongolian) and delivered using the Moodle 3.9 LMS, reaching both domestic and international students. By 2023, ICUMS supported over 16,000 students with 2,000 + multimedia materials and 493 professors.
This initiative demonstrates how localized digital infrastructure, pedagogical partnerships, and government policy alignment can scale equitable and ethically sound postgraduate training in emerging health systems.

Voices from the field – Mongolia

"I never imagined becoming a nurse – but after losing my aunt to late-diagnosed cancer, I chose this path to help prevent such losses for others."
One nurse with 15 years of experience in Mongolia reflected on her ethical awakening after attending a digital ethics course:
"We are not just assistants – we are advisors, educators, and human beings with our own struggles. But too often, our ethical voices are silenced by hierarchy and workload."
Her story underscores the need for inclusive, reflective ethics training that empowers all health professionals – not just physicians – to speak, be heard, and act ethically, even under pressure.

Box 5.
Online master's in Medical Sciences in Mongolia: Digital Innovation and Ethics.

highlight the ethical and structural challenges shaping Mongolia's digital health landscape:

5. Conclusion and future directions

The integration of medical ethics with digital and AI-driven technologies presents both unprecedented opportunities and complex dilemmas. As shown through Mongolian and global examples, the path forward requires intentional design: personalized pedagogy, secure and inclusive platforms, and ethical reflexivity embedded into every layer of medical education. Policymakers must ensure that digital ethics training is not optional but integrated into accreditation standards, CPD, and national health workforce strategies. Future research should evaluate the long-term outcomes of digital ethics interventions, exploring how competencies evolve over time and influence patient trust, system efficiency, and resilience in crisis contexts. By framing ethics as both a pedagogical and a policy priority, this chapter sets a forward-looking agenda for educators, regulators, and practitioners alike.

To succeed, institutions must:

- Prioritize ethical training alongside technological rollout;
- Codesign curricula with end-users, including patients;
- Establish oversight bodies (e.g., AI Ethics Boards); and
- Foster global-local dialog through shared case libraries and peer learning.

Ethical competence in the digital age is not optional – it is foundational to sustainable, equitable, and human-centered health care.

6. Expanding digital ethics in medical education: Directions and future priorities

6.1 Strengthening reflective digital practice

> *"Just as the golden sun nourishes all life indiscriminately, so too must a physician offer hope and uphold the dignity of every patient, regardless of their background or circumstances."*
>
> *One Mongolian doctor reflects on the sacred weight of medical ethics – not merely as a formal code, but as a lived commitment. For this physician, ethics transcend regulation:*
>
> *"To treat all patients with dignity, even in the face of death; to be present not merely with instruments, but with genuine compassion—this is the true essence of being a healer."*
>
> *This narrative illuminates the emotional resilience and high ethical standards required in life-and-death decisions, especially within culturally intimate and under-resourced environments.*

Medical ethics education must move beyond content delivery to cultivate digital self-awareness, ethical reflexivity, and judgment. Digital portfolios, interactive reflection tools, and AI-assisted feedback can support learners in evaluating their ethical growth over time. As illustrated in **Box 6**, emerging digital innovations in Mongolia's medical education system provide opportunities to embed ethics more deeply into training pathways.

As one Mongolian physician reflected:

> *"During my early clinical training, I inadvertently discussed a patient's sensitive test results in a public space. That moment profoundly transformed my understanding of medical ethics—from a superficial concern for professional appearance to a deep-seated respect for patient privacy, dignity, and empathy."*

Case box: Comparative insights in digital health

- **Global ranking**: Nations such as Norway, South Korea, and Iceland lead in digital health maturity; Mongolia ranks in Tier 3 out of 4.

- **Spending gap**: Health spending per capita is $10,921 in the United States vs. $163 in Mongolia (World Bank, 2022).

- **System efficiency**: WHO ranks Mongolia 145th out of 191 in health system efficiency – underscoring a need for strategic, ethical digital investment.

Real-life experiences from Mongolian clinicians highlight the urgency of ethical vigilance in high-pressure environments. As one physician reflected, "Ethics is not just about how we look or speak—it's about protecting patients' dignity when they're most vulnerable." This underscores the importance of reflective training in clinical ethics, particularly in digital and multicultural contexts.

The integration of medical ethics with digital and AI-driven technologies presents both unprecedented opportunities and complex dilemmas. As shown through Mongolian and global examples, the path forward requires intentional design: personalized pedagogy, secure and inclusive platforms, and ethical reflexivity embedded into every layer of medical education.
To succeed, institutions must:

- Prioritize ethical training alongside technological rollout;

- Codesign curricula with end-users, including patients;

- Establish oversight bodies (e.g., AI Ethics Boards); and

- Foster global-local dialog through shared case libraries and peer learning.

Ethical competence in the digital age is not optional – it is foundational to sustainable, equitable, and human-centered health care.

Box 6.
Digital health: Ethics and Global Lessons for Mongolia.

Such first-hand reflections highlight the importance of structured self-reflection in clinical education and underscore the necessity of cultivating digital self-awareness and ethical maturity from the earliest stages of training.

6.2 Scaling contextualized e-learning platforms

Mongolia's vast geography and sparse rural population present unique challenges to in-person training. According to the Ministry of Health (2022), over 50% of healthcare workers in Mongolia have expressed interest in e-learning opportunities. WHO further reports that, globally, 40% of healthcare staff lack adequate access to workplace-based training. In response, Mongolia has begun piloting online platforms and open-access digital resources tailored to

Clinical Communication Skills, offering flexible, scalable solutions especially valuable for professionals in remote areas. These platforms address both equity and quality, bridging training gaps without requiring relocation or service disruption.

MNUMS initiated pilot programs based on a learning-style needs assessment to address these gaps.

6.3 Embedding ethics into digital health policy

As Mongolia and other emerging economies scale national digital health systems, ethical dimensions must be integrated into technology rollouts. Digital health tools should include mechanisms for consent, accountability, and equitable access by design. Training must equip professionals to critically evaluate and navigate these frameworks [14].

6.4 Building a regional community of practice

To address common challenges in low- and middle-income countries, regional collaboration in ethics education should be expanded. Shared case repositories, multilingual content libraries, and collaborative research can foster resilience and innovation in digital ethics training.

6.5 Aligning with global digital transformation trends

Comparative analysis shows Mongolia falls within the “Emerging Economies” category in digital health transformation, alongside Brazil, Lebanon, and others. To progress, targeted investment in secure infrastructure, digital literacy, and instructional design is needed. Priorities should align with UN Sustainable Development Goals and WHO digital health frameworks.

6.6 Ethical implications of immersive technologies

Emerging technologies such as the metaverse offer immersive training environments for health professionals, enabling reflective practice, emotional intelligence development, and values-based decision-making through virtual reality simulations. However, these innovations raise concerns about psychological safety, data privacy, and the blurred boundaries between real and simulated identities. Institutions must proactively develop ethical guidelines for the use of such platforms, especially in preparing clinicians to care for displaced populations, postconflict communities, and culturally diverse patients.

7. Emerging innovations in ethics education

7.1 Gamified ethics learning

Gamification provides an engaging medium to explore ethical scenarios in low-risk, repeatable environments. Ethics “escape rooms,” scenario games, and decision-based progress challenges can stimulate critical thinking and peer collaboration. When learners solve ethical dilemmas in a game-based format, they demonstrate higher retention and emotional connection with the subject matter [14].

7.2 Blockchain in consent education

Blockchain technology can simulate real-world ethical processes such as informed consent. It enhances traceability, nonrepudiation, and accountability – critical in decentralized health systems and clinical trials. Blockchain empowers patients to manage their own data while ensuring that health professionals adhere to ethical consent protocols (Choi and Xu, 2022).

Author details

Omboosuren Bolorsaikhan[1*], Gelegjamts Delgersuren[2] and Gantulga Darambazar[3]

1 Department of Communication Skills, School of Bio-Medicine, Mongolian National University of Medical Sciences, Ulaanbaatar City, Mongolia

2 Head of Nursing Department, Medical School of Mongolian National University, Ulaanbaatar City, Mongolia

3 Mongolian National University of Medical Sciences, Ulaanbatar City, Mongolia

*Address all correspondence to: bolorsaikhan@mnums.edu.mn

References

[1] Russell SJ, Norvig P. Artificial Intelligence: A Modern Approach. 4th ed. Pearson; 2020. p. 10. https://lib.ysu.am/disciplines_bk/efdd4d1d4c2087fe1cbe03d9ced67f34.pdf

[2] Zhou Z-H. Machine Learning. Springer Nature; 2021. DOI: 10.1007/978-981-15-1967-3

[3] Russell SJ. Artificial Intelligence a Modern Approach. Pearson Education, Inc; 2010. https://repo.darmajaya.ac.id/5272/1/Artificial%20Intelligence-A%20Modern%20Approach%20(3rd%20Edition)%20(%20PDFDrive%20).pdf

[4] Montgomery KA. How Doctors Think: Clinical Judgment and the Practice of Medicine. Oxford University Press; 2006. https://global.oup.com/academic/product/how-doctors-think-9780195187120

[5] Foronda-Robles C, et al. The role of the web and social media in the tourism promotion of a world heri-tage site. The case of the Alcazar of Seville (Spain). Revista de Estudios Andaluces. 2021;**41**:47–64. DOI: 10.12795/rea.2021.i41.03

[6] Panahi O. AI ushering in a new era of digital dental medicine. Acta Scientific Medical Sciences. 2024;**8**(8). https://www.researchgate.net/publication/382397373

[7] Wang G, Badal A, Jia X, et al. Development of metaverse for intelligent healthcare. Nature Machine Intelligence. 2022;**4**:922–929. DOI: 10.1038/s42256-022-00549-6

[8] Subbiah V. The next generation of evidence-based medicine. Nature Medicine, 2023;**29**(1):49–58. DOI: 10.1038/s41591-022-02160-z

[9] Panahi1 O, Safaralizadeh R. How Artificial Intelligence and Biotechnology are Transforming Dentistry. 2024. https://juniperpublishers.com/aibm/pdf/AIBM.MS.ID.555981.pdf [Accessed: 2024-June-14]

[10] European Commission. Ethics guidelines for trustworthy AI. Availble from: https://digital-strategy.ec.europa.eu/en/library/ethics-guidelines-trustworthy-ai [Accessed: 2021-July-31]

[11] Retracted: Diagnostic Classification and Prognostic Prediction Using Common Genetic Variants in Autism Spectrum Disorder: Genotype-Based Deep Learning

[12] UNESCO. Ethics and Artificial Intelligence. 2021. https://unesdoc.unesco.org/ark:/48223/pf0000377250

[13] World Bank. Current Health Expenditure per Capita (Current US$). Availble from: https://data.worldbank.org/indicator/SH.XPD.CHEX.PC.CD [Accessed: 2022-December-31]

[14] World Health Organization. Global strategy on digital health. 2020–2025. Availble from: https://www.who.int/publications/i/item/9789240020924 [Accessed: 2023-December-31]

Chapter 10

Ethical Considerations and Informed Consent in the Use of Physical Restraints in Healthcare

Daisy Michelle Princeton, Gülendam Hakverdioğlu Yönt and Sezer Kisa

Abstract

The use of physical restraints in healthcare is a complex and ethically sensitive practice that requires carefully balancing patient safety with respect for autonomy, dignity, and fundamental human rights. While restraints can sometimes be necessary to prevent immediate harm, their use carries substantial risks, including physical injury, psychological distress, diminished freedom, loss of personal autonomy, social isolation, a sense of abandonment, and erosion of trust in the therapeutic relationship. This chapter critically examines the ethical principles underpinning decisions about physical restraint, including beneficence, non-maleficence, autonomy, and justice, and highlights the tensions that arise when these principles conflict. It emphasizes individualized clinical assessments, challenges around informed consent, the role of multidisciplinary decision-making, and practical strategies for resolving ethical dilemmas. Furthermore, it underscores the need for strict adherence to legal and institutional policies to safeguard patient rights and ensure accountability. By adopting a reflective and rights-based approach, healthcare professionals can minimize restraint use, uphold ethical standards, and foster a culture of care that prioritizes dignity, compassion, and patient-centered practice.

Keywords: physical restraint, ethical considerations, informed consent, ethical decision-making, legal principles, institutional guidelines

1. Introduction

Physical restraints (PRs) are widely used across healthcare settings worldwide, though their prevalence varies considerably by region, care context, and patient population. Reported rates range from 5% to 33% in general hospitals [1, 2], with the highest use seen in intensive care units and long-term care settings, where agitation affects up to 80% of patients and is often cited as justification for restraint [3–5]. Similarly, in psychiatric units, restraints are commonly used to prevent self-harm or aggression, while in nursing homes and other long-term care facilities, they are frequently applied to prevent falls or wandering among older adults with dementia

[6–9]. However, the use of PRs is often influenced more by culture, organizational structure, staffing levels, staff training [10], attitudes, and leadership than by the patient's actual clinical condition, reflecting systemic and training-related factors rather than genuine clinical necessity [11, 12]. This variability, which depends on patient circumstances, institutional practices, and country-specific contexts, highlights the need to critically examine the ethical, legal, and clinical frameworks that govern PR practices.

PR is generally defined as any device, material, or physical force used to prevent, restrict, or subdue a person's movement – either partially or completely – primarily to control behavior or ensure safety [10, 11]. Broader definitions also describe it as any action or device that limits an individual's ability to move freely or access their own body when it is attached to or placed near the body in a way the person cannot easily remove or control [12]. Examples include belts, wrist or ankle straps, vests, bed rails, chairs with fixed tables, or tightly tucked sheets that restrict mobility [6, 13]. PRs are distinct from chemical restraints, which involve the use of medications administered to control behavior or restrict movement, and from environmental restraints, which use architectural or environmental barriers, such as locked units, enclosed spaces, or seclusion rooms, to restrict freedom [14, 15]. This distinction is essential, as the ethical and clinical justifications for each form differ substantially, and conflating them can obscure the specific ethical challenges raised by PR.

Many factors contribute to the use of PRs, including institutional culture, service organization, staffing levels, and staff attitudes, which often influence their application more than the patient's clinical condition. Inadequate staffing and insufficient training can create environments where restraints are used as a default strategy rather than a last-resort intervention based on individualized clinical need. This highlights that restraint use is shaped as much by systemic and organizational factors as by patient-related ones, underscoring the importance of targeted interventions to shift institutional culture, improve training, and ensure adequate staffing to reduce unnecessary restraint use [7, 16–18]. A recent study highlighted that due to heavy workloads and overcrowded wards, staff often feel pressured to overlook patient rights and autonomy and resort to PR [19]. Although the literature consistently shows that staff generally hold negative attitudes toward the use of PR, they often apply it believing it to be necessary to protect patient safety [20], particularly to prevent incidents such as falls or the accidental removal of essential medical devices. However, as Jang et al. emphasized, the absence of clear criteria makes such decisions highly challenging and heavily reliant on individual clinical judgment [21].

Despite their frequent use, PRs remain one of the most ethically and legally contested interventions in healthcare. Although avoiding the use of PRs may carry some risk of physical harm – such as skin injuries and edema, nerve damage and ischemia, joint dislocation, vascular injury, and muscular pain and stiffness [19]; as well as psychological effects like fear, depression, anger, aggression, restlessness, agitation, and anxiety – recent literature indicates that their use ultimately causes more harm than benefit [7, 13, 17, 20, 22, 23]. Their application can also erode trust between patients and caregivers, undermining therapeutic relationships and the moral integrity of care environments [11, 19]. At the same time, healthcare professionals face ethical dilemmas as they try to balance patient autonomy with safety and fear legal repercussions if harm occurs, which can lead to emotional distress, self-doubt, and clinical misjudgment [5, 11]. From a human rights perspective, international frameworks, including the Universal Declaration of Human Rights (UDHR) [24], the European Convention on Human Rights (ECHR) [25], and the United Nations Convention on the Rights of Persons with Disabilities (UNCRPD) [26], emphasize autonomy, dignity, and freedom from degrading or inhumane treatment. Therefore, the World Health Organization (WHO) [27] and the Joint Commission on Accreditation of Healthcare Organizations [28] have called for minimizing and, where possible, eliminating coercive practices, including restraints, and for strengthening safeguards, documentation, and oversight.

Concerns about misuse, overuse, and challenges with PR have led to global calls for restraint reduction and the promotion of restraint-free care environments. Minimizing the use of PRs and, when their use is unavoidable, ensuring careful, time-limited, and standardized application while reducing the associated physical and psychosocial risks has become a stated priority in numerous patient safety guidelines [28]. International guidelines and recent studies suggest that restraint-free models of care with acceptable safety levels are feasible and that PR should not be used unless there is an immediate risk of serious harm [7, 16, 29]. The American Nurses Association (ANA) position statement, Reduction of Patient Restraint and Seclusion in Health Care Settings [30], recognized that restraints may sometimes be necessary but must only be used when "clinically appropriate" and "adequately justified." The International Psychogeriatric Association has expressed concern about the continued high prevalence and inappropriate use of PRs to manage neuropsychiatric symptoms in older people across both high- and low-to-middle-income countries [29]. Similarly, the National Bioethics Committee in Italy concluded that restraints should be used only as a last resort in situations of genuine and imminent danger, applied proportionally and for the shortest necessary time, and never solely due to agitation or once the risk has passed [16].

2. Ethical foundation of PR use

The ethical foundation of using PR is grounded in the obligation to protect patient safety while simultaneously respecting autonomy, dignity, and fundamental human rights. Because PRs inherently restrict personal freedom, their use requires rigorous ethical justification and must be regarded as a measure of last resort. Deciding whether to use restraints often creates ethical dilemmas, as healthcare professionals must weigh the risks and benefits while balancing patient safety with respect for autonomy. Therefore, decisions about restraint use should be guided by the core bioethical principles that underpin all healthcare practice: autonomy, beneficence, non-maleficence, and justice, ensuring that clinical actions protect safety while safeguarding dignity, preserving rights, and promoting equitable care.

The stated purpose of PR is to "protect" and "control." However, while restraints may be intended to prevent harm to patients or others, they inevitably limit the free will of those subjected to them, particularly psychiatric or cognitively impaired patients, thereby placing their basic human rights at risk [5, 31]. Applying restraints in the name of safety not only exposes patients to potential physical and psychological harm but also raises profound ethical concerns about the value placed on the autonomy and dignity of individuals with unique identities. Because both patient safety and patient autonomy are fundamental rights that must be ethically protected, healthcare professionals must carefully balance these principles rather than prioritizing one at the expense of the other.

The ethical debate surrounding PR is further framed in the Hippocratic maxim of "first, do no harm," which obliges clinicians to prevent harm while avoiding practices that may compromise rights or dignity [32]. Ethical practice requires transparency, robust informed consent procedures, and meticulous documentation of restraint use and its alternatives. Any use of restraints without valid consent or without consideration of less restrictive measures represents a breach of professional standards, human rights obligations, and legal duties and must be actively addressed within healthcare systems.

Building on this ethical foundation, the following sections examine the four core bioethical principles – autonomy, beneficence, non-maleficence, and justice – as they relate to PR use in healthcare. These principles provide a structured framework for navigating the ethical tensions that arise when protecting patients from harm requires actions that limit their freedom. By critically exploring how each principle applies in practice, this chapter aims to support healthcare professionals in making ethically sound, legally compliant, and patient-centered decisions about the use of PR.

2.1 Autonomy

The principle of autonomy emphasizes respect for individuals' moral self-determination, ensuring that their preferences and values guide decisions about their care, even in conditions of dependency. As a cornerstone of biomedical ethics, autonomy affirms each person's right to make informed choices regarding their own care. Upholding a person's autonomy and dignity is widely regarded as a fundamental prerequisite for effective therapeutic care [16]. As Dworkin [33] argues, autonomy represents both the right and the capacity of individuals to govern their own lives according to values they have chosen for themselves, making it a foundational principle for ethical healthcare practice. In the context of PR, this principle is especially challenged because restraints restrict personal freedom and decision-making capacity [5]. Respecting autonomy requires that patients are involved in decisions about their care wherever possible, and that their preferences, values, and previously expressed wishes are honored. Sometimes a patient's right to make their own choices can conflict with a clinician's duty of beneficence, creating a dilemma over whether the clinician's main duty is to prioritize the patient's well-being or to respect their autonomy. This underscores that the very role of healthcare providers rests on offering interventions that actively enhance patients' health, and therefore the patient's preferences should always be considered, with decisions about restraint use involving the patient and caregivers as early as possible in the process [7]. Any decision to limit patient autonomy must be justified by clear evidence of imminent harm, implemented using the least restrictive means available, and accompanied by comprehensive documentation of the decision-making process in the patient's record.

At the heart of Western moral philosophy lies the conviction that individuals possess an inalienable right to self-determination and bodily autonomy [33, 34], and physically restraining patients represents a substantial infringement on a person's liberty and bodily integrity, potentially violating this autonomy [13, 35]. However, in many situations, individuals may lack the capacity to provide informed consent, necessitating the involvement of a legal proxy [36, 37]. As with all healthcare procedures, informed consent is essential and applies equally to the use of PRs, except in true emergencies where it may be temporarily waived. PR must not be applied to mentally competent individuals without their consent, as it violates core principles of autonomy and human rights [35–37]. Even when cognitive impairment is present, individuals should be involved in decision-making as much as possible, with caregivers and relatives considering the person's likely wishes. If no legal guardian is available, decisions about PR should be made by the multidisciplinary team based on the option that offers the greatest benefit to the person [36]. Ethically, even if a patient is attempting to remove medical devices, PR should not be applied without consent, as the act itself constitutes a significant restriction of personal liberty [13, 20, 36]. In such cases, alternative measures should be considered. For instance, for individuals with impaired cognitive function, such as dementia or Alzheimer's disease, bed rails should only be used after less restrictive options, such as lowering the bed height [13], placing a mattress on the floor [13], or using surveillance technology such as acoustic and visual monitoring systems, door sensors, and infrared bed or chair sensors [38], have been attempted.

2.2 Beneficence and non-maleficence

The principle of beneficence emphasizes safeguarding the integrity of the person by acting with beneficial intent, avoiding harm, and promoting health, social integration, and participation for individuals in vulnerable situations. Non-maleficence involves avoiding harm, preventing potential harm, removing existing harm, and promoting good. Together, the ethical principles of beneficence and non-maleficence form a cornerstone of healthcare practice and are especially significant in discussions about PR. Beneficence obligates healthcare professionals to actively promote patient well-being [39], prevent harm, and take positive actions to improve health outcomes, while non-maleficence requires them to refrain from actions that could cause harm [34, 39]. These principles are often cited to justify the use of PRs, which are perceived as protective measures to prevent self-injury, falls, or interference with life-sustaining treatment [19, 40]. However, growing evidence increasingly questions this reasoning, showing that restraints often cause more harm than benefit [11, 20].

As previously mentioned, the harms associated with PR are well-documented and multifaceted. Physically, restraint use has been linked to bruises, skin tears, fractures, contractures, reduced mobility, pressure ulcers, and even death through asphyxiation or strangulation [22, 41, 42]. Psychologically, it can induce fear, humiliation, anger, distress, agitation, emotional resignation, and post-traumatic stress, while also contributing to cognitive decline [7, 11]. These consequences directly conflict with the principle of non-maleficence, as an act intended to protect the patient paradoxically inflicts significant harm.

Decision-making about PR is ethically complex, requiring healthcare professionals to weigh potential short-term safety benefits against the substantial physical and psychological harms documented in the literature. Healthcare professionals must balance competing duties, such as protecting safety or managing disruptive behavior, while respecting autonomy, dignity, and emotional well-being, often in high-pressure situations requiring rapid judgment. Ideally, they should weigh the potential short-term benefits, such as preventing a fall or removing a medical device, against substantial long-term physical and psychological harms

[43]. Goethals et al. [11] emphasized that many nurses acknowledged the importance of preserving patients' freedom of movement and dignity, even in complex clinical situations [11]; however, studies show that time constraints, heavy workloads, and institutional cultures often skew decision-making toward risk avoidance rather than ethical reflection [5, 17, 44]. In practice, this can result in the principle of autonomy being overridden, and informed consent is frequently unobtainable. Nurses may justify prioritizing perceived safety over patient choice, comfort, and emotional integrity [19, 20, 40, 42]. This reflects an ethically problematic shift in which beneficence is interpreted narrowly as physical protection, while its broader intent — promoting overall well-being — is overlooked.

This ethical tension is further complicated by misconceptions about the effectiveness of restraints. Importantly, several recent studies indicate that staff often overestimate the protective benefits of restraints while underestimating their risks. Studies have found that restraint use does not reliably prevent falls among older adults in acute care [6, 45], while Sharifi et al. [22] reported that patients subjected to restraints were more likely to experience functional decline and institutionalization. These findings challenge the assumption that restraint is an effective safety intervention and reinforce the argument that its harm often outweighs its intended benefits. Moreover, the impact of restraint can extend beyond the patient to diminish staff morale [9, 46] and undermine the overall ethical climate within care environments [19]. Goethals et al. [11] reported that nurses who used restraints experienced moral distress, guilt, and ethical conflict, highlighting that even perceived beneficence carries moral costs to staff and the therapeutic relationship [11].

The principles of beneficence and non-maleficence require that PRs be used only as an absolute last resort, after all less restrictive alternatives have been attempted and documented. When their use becomes unavoidable, it must be continuously evaluated to ensure that the intended benefits outweigh potential harm, with regular reassessment, close monitoring, and prompt removal once the risk has passed. Without these ethical safeguards, restraints risk undermining not only patient safety but also the core values of healthcare. Applying PRs without clear justification, valid consent, and ongoing oversight is increasingly seen as incompatible with human rights obligations, putting dignity, autonomy, and equality at risk [7, 47]. This human rights-based perspective is reflected in principles outlined by the Australian Evidence-Based Healthcare Centre (2013), which include three core principles for restraint use: avoid using restraints whenever possible, remove them as soon as they are no longer needed, and seek alternative methods whenever feasible [5]. Embedding these human rights principles into everyday practice is essential to ensure care remains both ethical and legally sound, as restraint use – except when safety is a legitimate concern – can conflict with the very principles of beneficence and non-maleficence.

2.3 Justice

Justice is a fundamental ethical principle that demands fairness, equity, and impartiality in the provision of healthcare. In the context of PR, it requires healthcare professionals to make decisions that are free from discrimination or bias, ensuring that all patients are treated with equal respect and dignity. This principle extends beyond individual interactions to encompass systemic fairness, meaning that institutional policies, staffing levels, and resource allocation practices must not create conditions where restraints are used disproportionately on vulnerable populations, such as older adults, individuals with dementia, or socially marginalized groups.

Upholding justice necessitates the consistent application of ethical standards, transparency in decision-making, and robust accountability mechanisms to prevent inequitable or arbitrary use of restraints. When justice is overlooked, restraint practices risk reinforcing existing health disparities and undermining the ethical integrity of care. Justice complements autonomy, beneficence, and non-maleficence by emphasizing fairness, equity, and the equal moral worth of all individuals. In this context, justice requires healthcare professionals to exercise prudent judgment and avoid unnecessary risks [42], ensuring that decisions to use restraints are not only clinically justified and ethically sound but also applied consistently without discrimination or bias. It further demands that vulnerable populations, such as frail older adults or individuals with cognitive impairment, are not subjected to restraints solely because of their vulnerability or for the convenience of staff [16].

Justice also encompasses the fair distribution of institutional resources. It requires that the use of restraints does not stem from systemic shortcomings, such as understaffing, inadequate training, or lack of supportive infrastructure, which compromise ethical care [17]. Inadequate knowledge or training can lead to inconsistent or biased application, resulting in inequitable treatment of vulnerable populations, particularly older adults, individuals with dementia, and patients from marginalized social groups [16, 38]. This raises concerns about discriminatory practices and systemic injustice within healthcare settings.

Justice becomes particularly complex when patients are detained for public safety, as the focus shifts from individual rights to protecting others. In a system that undervalues and underfunds mental health care, restraints are often used unfairly because the staff best equipped to build therapeutic relationships are scarce, leading to unequal treatment and violating the principle of justice [48].

All patients must receive fair and equitable treatment regardless of their vulnerabilities. This principle is especially relevant in the context of PRs, as frail older adults and other marginalized groups must not be disproportionately or unjustly subjected to restraint. Using restraints for staff convenience, due to understaffing, or as a "quick fix" to manage challenging behaviors is widely regarded as ethically and morally unacceptable. Such practices prioritize institutional efficiency over patient rights and dignity, thereby violating the principle of justice [5]. Because justice depends not only on individual actions but also on the ethical culture of the workplace, ensuring a supportive environment is essential to preventing unjust restraint practices. Creating conditions where staff are supported, protected, and ethically empowered is therefore part of upholding justice in care. According to the ANA's position statement, Provision 6 of the Code of Ethics highlights nurses' responsibility to establish, maintain, and improve the ethical environment of their workplace, a duty that is especially important for nurse managers and executives [49].

3. Informed consent as an ethical foundation of healthcare practice

The principle of informed consent, grounded in the ethical values of autonomy and self-determination, requires the disclosure of relevant information, a voluntary decision, and sufficient decision-making capacity [50]. It is central to ethically sound care delivery and is widely recognized as a cornerstone of patient autonomy, which itself underpins basic human rights [51]. Informed consent affirms that individuals hold the moral right to make informed decisions about their own bodies and healthcare. Informed consent is often treated as just paperwork, but simply handing patients a form is not enough. It should be a meaningful, two-way conversation between providers and those giving consent, not a one-time event [50]. Healthcare professionals must inform individuals of potential risks and benefits of PR, and patients must be able to ask questions and voice concerns before deciding whether to consent. However, in cases of cognitive impairment, patients' ability to comprehend and evaluate treatment options may be limited.

The use of PRs without valid consent constitutes a direct violation of these rights, undermining autonomy, dignity, and self-respect [22, 51–53]. Seeking and obtaining informed consent is, therefore, a critical mechanism for upholding these inherent rights and ensuring justice in care delivery. Nevertheless, tensions often arise between respecting autonomy and ensuring safety, particularly when a patient's decision could place themselves or others at risk [54]. Personal autonomy is not absolute; it must not endanger others' rights and can only be meaningfully exercised when the individual has adequate decision-making capacity [47].

Informed consent obligates providers to give patients, their legal proxies, or relatives full, comprehensible information about their condition; treatment options; potential risks, benefits, and side effects [22, 52]. Such transparency enables patients or their legal representatives to weigh the potential benefits of restraint against its risks, thereby helping to prevent harm and promote good outcomes [51, 52]. Improper use of restraints, particularly without valid consent, has been associated with severe adverse outcomes [22, 37, 53]. These consequences represent a clear failure of just care. Healthcare professionals must, therefore, carefully balance the advantages and disadvantages of restraint to reach an ethically sound decision [5]. In practice, however, autonomy is often constrained, especially when obtaining consent is impossible, while beneficence and non-maleficence are used to justify prioritizing safety over freedom, comfort, or emotional well-being.

3.1 Addressing vulnerabilities and diminished capacity

Justice also requires that the rights of individuals with diminished decision-making capacity, such as those with cognitive impairment or dementia, be fully protected [51]. In such cases, informed consent must be sought from a legal proxy, substitute decision-maker, or family member [7, 22, 51–53]. Some national legislation, such as Norway's Patient Rights Act, explicitly mandates documentation of failed alternative interventions before restraints can be applied to individuals lacking decision-making capacity, reinforcing a commitment to person-centered care [55]. In line with ethical principles, informed consent discussions must include the purpose of restraint, its potential risks (non-maleficence), benefits (beneficence), and possible alternatives, while allowing adequate opportunities for questions and review. For individuals unable to provide consent, this process should be carried out with their legal representative or proxy [29]. Fields and Calvert concluded that evaluating the capacity of patients with cognitive impairment to understand treatment options is vital for essential informed consent and should be guided by established best practices [50].

DOI: http://dx.doi.org/10.5772/intechopen.1013160

3.2 Promoting accountability and ethical professional conduct

Informed consent is embedded within ethical and legal frameworks and should be reinforced through clear, standardized institutional policies [7, 52, 53]. Consistent application of informed consent procedures reduces uncertainty, prevents unjust or arbitrary use of restraints, and upholds professional accountability. Failure to obtain consent can result in professional, legal, and ethical repercussions and contribute to moral distress among staff [22, 52]. Nurses have acknowledged that restraining patients without consent constitutes a violation of human rights [52]. Upholding informed consent, therefore, promotes accountability, aligns practice with ethical and legal standards, and serves as a mechanism for ensuring justice in care.

Despite its critical importance, obtaining valid informed consent faces practical challenges. Healthcare providers may bypass consent due to fear of patient or family refusal, concerns about conflict, or perceptions that the process is too time-consuming in busy environments [52]. Some nurses remain unaware that formal permission is required or that procedures exist for obtaining it [52]. While family consent is essential for patients lacking capacity, some studies suggest that family-signed permissions may inadvertently increase restraint use by alleviating the moral and legal pressure felt by staff [40]. These findings highlight that achieving justice through informed consent requires sustained commitment, ongoing staff education, and strict adherence to policies that prioritize patients' rights, preferences, and well-being [51].

3.3 Barriers to obtaining informed consent

While informed consent is central to ensuring justice, its consistent implementation in real-world clinical settings remains challenging. Numerous barriers can hinder the proper acquisition of valid consent. The use of PRs in vulnerable individuals, particularly within nursing homes and hospital settings, further underscores these challenges, as it raises complex ethical, legal, and clinical dilemmas surrounding informed consent. Obtaining valid informed consent is both a legal and ethical duty, central to upholding patient autonomy and safeguarding human rights; however, in practice, this obligation is frequently overlooked, inconsistently applied, or poorly documented, creating serious ethical and legal concerns.

Barriers to obtaining informed consent for PR use can be broadly grouped into patient-related, staff-related, and systemic or institutional factors. Patient-related barriers often include cognitive impairment, delirium, dementia, communication difficulties, or acute distress, which may compromise the person's decision-making capacity and ability to understand or retain information. Staff-related barriers involve inadequate knowledge of ethical and legal requirements, limited skills in consent communication, time pressures, fear of patient or family refusal, and a prevailing belief that consent is unnecessary when safety is at stake. Systemic barriers include insufficient staffing levels, high workload, lack of clear institutional guidelines or standardized consent procedures, poor documentation systems, and organizational cultures that normalize restraint use as routine care. These barriers often intersect, creating conditions where restraints are applied without valid consent, undermining patient autonomy and violating ethical and legal standards.

In rare emergency situations where there is an immediate threat of serious harm to the patient or others, PRs may be applied without prior informed consent as a temporary protective measure. However, such exceptions must be strictly time-limited, continuously reassessed, and used only until the immediate danger subsides. Comprehensive documentation is essential in these cases to ensure accountability and legal compliance. Records should include the clinical justification for restraint, the specific emergency circumstances, the type and duration of restraint used, the alternatives attempted, continuous monitoring notes, and a post-event debriefing with staff, the patient, and their family or proxy decision-maker [7, 47]. This documentation safeguards patient rights, facilitates review, and helps prevent inappropriate normalization of emergency restraint use.

3.3.1 Patient-related barriers

Patient-related factors are among the most common challenges to obtaining valid informed consent for PR use. Older adults, particularly those in hospitals or long-term care settings, often experience cognitive impairment, dementia, delirium, or acute confusion that compromises their decision-making capacity [7]. Communication difficulties, sensory deficits such as hearing or vision loss, language barriers, and emotional distress can further limit their ability to comprehend information or express preferences [56]. In such circumstances, patients may be unable to understand the purpose, risks, or alternatives to restraint, making it difficult to obtain truly informed consent. Although legal frameworks typically require the use of proxy or legal representative decision-makers when capacity is lacking, in practice, these representatives are not always available, consulted, or adequately informed, leaving patients vulnerable to being restrained without proper consent [7, 52].

3.3.2 Staff-related barriers

Barriers also stem from staff knowledge, attitudes, and working conditions. Many healthcare professionals receive limited or no formal training on the ethical and legal requirements of obtaining consent for restraints, leading to uncertainty or misconceptions about when and how consent should be sought. High workload, time pressures, and stressful clinical environments may discourage staff from engaging in time-consuming consent discussions, especially during emergencies or periods of patient agitation. Some nurses fear that seeking consent may provoke patient or family refusal, conflict, or anger, while others believe that patients will not understand or will refuse consent regardless [57]. In some settings, there is also a prevailing perception that safety needs override the need for consent, resulting in restraints being applied as a default protective measure rather than as a last resort after informed agreement [37]. These staff-related factors contribute to a culture in which obtaining informed consent is undervalued or bypassed, undermining patient autonomy and ethical care standards.

Effective communication is crucial when seeking informed consent or explaining restraint use to vulnerable groups, such as individuals with dementia, delirium, sensory impairments, or language barriers. Tailored strategies include using simple, clear language; visual aids; repetition; and allowing extra time for processing information [29]. Involving interpreters or culturally competent staff is essential for patients with limited language proficiency to ensure understanding and respect for cultural values. For those with cognitive impairment, engaging family members or legal proxies early in discussions, while still including the patient to the extent possible, promotes shared decision-making and preserves autonomy [6]. Such person-centered communication reduces confusion, distress, and resistance, while supporting ethical and informed decision-making.

3.3.3 Systemic and institutional barriers

Systemic and organizational factors also play a significant role in undermining the informed consent process. Chronic understaffing [21], inadequate skill mix, and heavy workloads can push institutions toward expedient practices, where restraints are used to manage behavior or reduce workload rather than out of clinical necessity. Many facilities lack clear institutional policies or standardized procedures outlining when and how to obtain consent for restraints, and documentation systems are often inconsistent or incomplete [6]. Furthermore, organizational cultures that normalize the routine use of restraints may discourage ethical reflection and reinforce the belief that consent is optional [37]. These systemic gaps weaken accountability mechanisms and contribute to the persistence of restraint use without valid informed consent, perpetuating violations of patient autonomy and human rights [7]. Understanding and addressing these barriers is essential for developing interventions that support ethical decision-making, strengthen consent practices, and ultimately protect vulnerable patients.

4. Challenges with informed consent in PR use

Key challenges related to obtaining informed consent for the use of PR are summarized in **Table 1**. The following subsections provide further explanations for each category.

Informed consent is a fundamental requirement for all health interventions, including the use of PR; yet, obtaining it is often challenging.

Key problems	Description
Absence or invalid consent processes [7, 57, 58]	Consent is often not obtained, is poorly documented, or is obtained through blanket authorizations rather than specific, informed discussions. Consent is sometimes sought only after restraints are applied.
Ethical and legal violations [16, 34, 36, 47]	Applying restraints without valid consent violates autonomy, dignity, and human rights, contradicts ethical and legal standards, and exposes staff/institutions to liability.
Moral distress and ethical conflict among staff [11, 19, 37, 44]	Bypassing consent causes nurses to experience guilt, emotional strain, and ethical conflict, undermining professional integrity and well-being.
Systemic accountability failures [6, 7]	Weak policies, poor documentation, and lack of oversight prevent quality monitoring and perpetuate unconsented restraint practices.

Table 1.
Key challenges related to obtaining informed consent for the use of PR.

4.1 Absence or invalid consent processes

A major concern in the use of PRs is the frequent absence or invalidity of informed consent procedures. Restraints are often applied without formal consent, with documentation missing or incomplete [7, 57]. In some facilities, "blanket authorizations," generic forms signed at admission, replace specific, time-limited consent for each restraint episode [58, 59]. Consent is sometimes sought only after restraints are applied or solely from legal representatives without involving the patient, contradicting ethical standards [58, 60]. Regulatory gaps further contribute to inconsistency, as some regions lack clear policies or legislation [6, 59]. These practices undermine essential safeguards, compromise patient autonomy, and place individuals at risk of harm.

Patient-related barriers compound the problem. Cognitive impairments such as dementia, delirium, or acute confusion often limit decision-making capacity [56, 59]. Yet, capacity is sometimes wrongly presumed absent solely due to a dementia diagnosis, excluding individuals who may have lucid intervals and retain the right to accept or refuse treatment [29, 34, 61]. When patients lack capacity, families may be involved in consent decisions, but this process is often unclear and lacks adequate information on restraint risks, benefits, and alternatives. Atee et al. [29] recommend a collaborative, team-based approach involving the patient whenever possible, together with proxies and interdisciplinary staff, to uphold autonomy, beneficence, non-maleficence, and safety [29]. Such shared decision-making promotes transparency, reduces bias, and strengthens ethical accountability [7].

4.2 Ethical and legal violations

Applying PRs without valid informed consent constitutes a serious breach of ethical and legal standards. It violates fundamental principles of autonomy, dignity, and human rights [34, 47]. In practice, consent is often sought only after restraints are applied or obtained solely from a representative without first attempting to involve the patient. Most legal frameworks require written consent for procedures that pose significant risks, including restraint use. Even when restraints are clinically indicated for patients with severe cognitive impairment or psychiatric conditions, informed consent must still be obtained from legally designated representatives [29, 57]. Regulatory gaps and unclear institutional policies worsen these problems, as many staff remain uncertain about consent requirements or unaware that formal procedures exist [6, 7, 62].

Multiple factors contribute to bypassing informed consent, including prioritizing safety over autonomy, staff convenience, and fear of litigation [1, 6, 59, 63–69]. Yet evidence shows that restraints may increase rather than reduce fall risk and legal liability [64, 69, 70]. Using restraints without consent constitutes an unequivocal violation of autonomy and a fundamental breach of human rights and freedom [68, 71, 72], often leaving patients feeling infantilized and stripped of control [64, 73]. Crutchfield [36] asserts that restraint without consent is a moral wrong and an impermissible violation of liberty [36]. They also cause moral distress and ethical conflict among staff [19, 40, 44, 74], while poor documentation undermines accountability and increases providers' vulnerability to malpractice claims [22, 51, 52].

Cognitive impairment further complicates the process of obtaining valid consent, as patients with dementia, delirium, or acute confusion may struggle to understand information or participate meaningfully in decision-making [6, 56, 64, 75, 76]. However, capacity is often wrongly presumed absent, excluding individuals who may experience lucid periods and retain the right to refuse treatment if adequately informed [29, 34, 61, 77]. When patients lack decision-making capacity, it is often incorrectly presumed absent; family consent may not reflect their values, especially when there is limited awareness of restraint risks or alternatives [55, 64, 70, 76, 78]. To address these gaps, best practice guidance emphasizes the need for clear legal definitions and policies for restraint use, comprehensive staff education on ethical and legal responsibilities, meticulous documentation, and regular audits [7, 18, 22, 61, 63, 66, 79]. Interdisciplinary, shared decision-making and a person-centered care model are also essential to reduce restraint use and safeguard patient autonomy, dignity, and human rights [7, 29, 51, 62].

4.3 Moral distress and ethical conflict among staff

Bypassing informed consent when using PRs often generates profound moral distress and ethical conflict among healthcare staff, particularly nurses. Salehi et al. [19] found that nurses in critical care settings experienced intense emotional strain, guilt, and inner conflict when they felt compelled to restrain patients without consent, perceiving this as a violation of patients' dignity and rights [19]. Similarly, Goethals et al. [11] reported that nurses struggled to reconcile their duty to ensure patient safety with their professional and ethical commitment to respect autonomy, often describing the decision to restrain as morally troubling and personally distressing [11]. De Casterlé et al. [44] highlighted how contextual pressures, such as institutional expectations, heavy workloads, and fear of adverse outcomes, can override ethical reflection, leading nurses to prioritize risk avoidance over patient-centered values [44]. Collectively, these studies underscore that bypassing consent not only harms patients but also undermines the moral and psychological well-being of healthcare professionals tasked with their care. Addressing this moral distress requires institutional support systems, ethics training, and clear policies that empower staff to prioritize patient rights while maintaining safety.

These challenges also carry legal and systemic implications. Healthcare providers and organizations face potential legal consequences, including negligence or malpractice claims, when restraints are used inappropriately or without valid informed consent [15, 42, 43]. Poor or absent documentation of restraint use and consent, often driven by fear of legal repercussions, further undermines accountability, obstructs quality evaluation, and impedes efforts to implement practice improvements [15]. Collectively, these physical, psychological, ethical, and legal harms reinforce that restraints should only ever be used as a last resort, after all reasonable alternatives have been exhausted and for the shortest possible duration.

4.4 Systemic accountability failures

Systemic accountability failures are a major factor enabling the continued use of PRs without valid informed consent. Weak or absent institutional policies, inadequate documentation practices, and insufficient managerial oversight create environments where restraint use goes largely unchecked, and ethical breaches remain concealed. Yönt et al. [6] reported that inadequate policy frameworks and minimal supervision in nursing homes contributed to highly variable restraint practices, often shaped more by organizational culture than by patient need [6]. Scheepmans et al. [7] highlighted that poor documentation of consent and restraint episodes obstructs audits, quality improvement efforts, and external accountability [7]. Low documentation rates make it difficult to evaluate the appropriateness of restraint use or to identify training needs, thereby perpetuating unsafe and unethical practices. Collectively, these findings demonstrate that without strong policies, clear procedures, and systematic oversight, healthcare organizations fail to detect or correct inappropriate restraint use, allowing violations of patient rights to persist unchecked.

5. Ethical decision-making models for PR use

Decisions about using PRs often arise in urgent, emotionally charged clinical contexts where staff must weigh competing ethical duties: protecting patient safety while preserving autonomy, dignity, and rights. To navigate these dilemmas, structured ethical decision-making models are essential for promoting consistency, transparency, and accountability in practice. Two widely recognized frameworks, the principlist approach and the four-quadrant approach, are particularly useful for guiding restraint-related decisions in healthcare.

The principlist model, articulated by Beauchamp and Childress [34], provides a foundational ethical framework based on four core bioethical principles: autonomy, beneficence, non-maleficence, and justice. This model requires clinicians to systematically evaluate: (1) whether the patient has decision-making capacity and their expressed preferences (autonomy); (2) whether the intervention is likely to benefit the patient (beneficence); (3) whether it poses risks or harms that could outweigh potential benefits (non-maleficence); and (4) whether its use would be fair, equitable, and non-discriminatory (justice).

Applying these principles compels clinicians to exhaust less-restrictive alternatives first, justify restraint use as a last resort, and document a clear rationale showing that the benefits substantially outweigh the risks [7, 22]. However, the principlist approach, although widely used, has notable limitations, as conflicting principles, time pressures, and risk-averse cultures can lead to superficial use, and its strong focus on autonomy makes it difficult to apply with patients lacking decision-making capacity. Practitioners should therefore use it cautiously and consider alternative approaches when autonomy is limited.

The four-quadrant (or four-box) model, originally developed by Jonsen, Siegler, and Winslade (2015), offers a more case-based structure by organizing ethical reasoning into four domains: medical indications, patient preferences, quality of life, and contextual features. This framework prompts multidisciplinary teams to consider: (1) the clinical indications, expected outcomes, and proportionality of restraint use; (2) the patient's values, preferences, or advance directives; (3) how restraint may affect the patient's quality of life, dignity, and psychological well-being; and (4) broader contextual issues, including legal regulations, institutional policies, cultural norms, and resource constraints. In practice, this model has been shown to reduce reliance on restraints by facilitating interdisciplinary dialog, balancing safety with autonomy, and ensuring that decisions are well-justified and ethically defensible [11]. It functions as a practical tool to identify and organize morally relevant issues but still requires additional ethical reasoning, such as combining it with the principlist model through specification and balancing, to guide final decisions. Studies using this approach suggest that it improves clarity and structure in complex ethical cases, and aligning it with the principlist model can help practitioners apply core ethical principles more consistently while addressing the specific contextual features of each case [80, 81].

Integrating these complementary models into institutional policies can support more consistent ethical decision-making, reduce moral uncertainty, and strengthen accountability in restraint practices, ultimately fostering a rights-based care culture that prioritizes patient dignity and preserves the ethical integrity of healthcare practice.

6. Approaches to minimizing PRs and managing ethical dilemmas

To address the ethical, legal, and clinical challenges surrounding PR use, several key recommendations have been proposed in the literature. A central principle is that restraints should be applied only as a measure of last resort – used solely when all reasonable, less restrictive alternatives have been exhausted, and then only for the shortest duration necessary [22, 51, 52]. This approach aims to minimize harm, preserve patient autonomy, and uphold ethical standards of care. Building on this principle, five main domains of action have been identified to transform current practices and strengthen safeguards against misuse.

6.1 Policy, regulation, and documentation

There is broad consensus on the need for a universal definition of PR to enable consistent reporting, regulation, and evaluation across settings [63, 66, 82]. Institutions should establish clear, evidence-based policies specifying indications, permissible duration, observation requirements, and review procedures, with regular updates [61, 73]. Strengthening legal and regulatory frameworks is also critical to ensure safe and ethical practices, incorporating both punitive measures for misuse and positive legislative support for alternative strategies [6, 18, 48, 79]. Meticulous documentation of rationale, consent process, application, monitoring, and review is essential for transparency, accountability, and auditability [7, 22, 52].

6.2 Education, training, and culture change

Comprehensive education for all healthcare staff and accessible information for patients and families are vital to raise awareness of the ethical implications, legal responsibilities, and risks of restraint [6, 55, 67, 73, 78, 83, 84]. Training should emphasize the availability and efficacy of alternative approaches while equipping staff with practical skills to implement restraint-free strategies safely and confidently, with a focus on recognizing and responding to the individual needs and behaviors of residents with cognitive impairments through person-centered care approaches. Evidence shows that targeted programs can significantly reduce restraint use, improve knowledge, and shift attitudes toward less restrictive care [62]. Sustained culture change requires visible leadership commitment, role models or "change champions," and ongoing feedback mechanisms [6, 22, 45].

6.3 Prioritizing alternatives and adequate resourcing

A "restraint-free" model should be actively promoted, where restraints are used only as a last resort when benefits clearly outweigh risks and no other viable options remain [13, 63, 75, 84, 85]. Implementing this model requires individualized care planning, proactive risk reduction, environmental modifications, and supportive interventions. Adequate staffing levels and investment in alternative approaches are essential, as understaffing is one of the strongest predictors of restraint use [7, 22, 53, 62]. Providing resources and supportive infrastructure is critical to achieving sustainable reductions.

6.4 Interdisciplinary and shared decision-making

Decisions about restraint use should involve physicians, nurses, and allied health professionals and, where possible, the patient and their family, with attention to advance care directives [18, 67, 73]. Enhancing collaboration and communication is also essential. Interdisciplinary care teams, ethics committees, and legal or proxy decision-makers should be actively involved in shared decision-making, while transparent documentation and open communication with patients and families are crucial to fostering trust and supporting informed participation. Such collaboration helps ensure that decisions are holistic, ethically sound, and aligned with patient values. From the outset, teams should promote open communication, shared responsibility, and transparent documentation throughout the decision-making process.

6.5 Monitoring, auditing, and person-centered care

Ongoing managerial oversight, regular audits, and continuous quality improvement are necessary to ensure adherence to guidelines and identify deviations [22, 51]. The absence of routine auditing has been linked to continued unconsented restraint use [7]. Embedding a person-centered care philosophy is equally crucial, prioritizing autonomy, dignity, and individual preferences over institutional convenience [51]. Implementing these policy recommendations can help healthcare professionals foster a safe, supportive, and person-centered environment that protects the rights and preserves the dignity of individuals in vulnerable situations.

7. Conclusion

The use of PRs remains one of the most profound ethical challenges in healthcare, requiring a careful balance between safeguarding patient safety and preserving autonomy, dignity, and fundamental human rights. This chapter has outlined the core ethical principles, informed consent requirements, legal mandates, and practical decision-making frameworks that must guide restraint practices. Future efforts must prioritize patient-centered and rights-based care by strengthening informed consent processes, fostering interdisciplinary collaboration, and investing in effective, restraint-free alternatives. Ethical and legal accountability should remain central to all policies, clinical guidelines, and research on PRs.

Ethical decision-making regarding restraint use must be grounded in the four foundational bioethical principles: autonomy, beneficence, non-maleficence, and justice. These principles require that PRs be used only as a last resort, after exhausting all less restrictive alternatives and ensuring that potential benefits clearly outweigh potential harms. Healthcare teams and organizations should work collaboratively to establish a restraint-free culture by embedding evidence-based alternatives into practice, prioritizing less restrictive measures, and enforcing robust multidisciplinary monitoring and oversight of any restraint use. In parallel, robust legal frameworks – spanning international human rights instruments such as the UDHR, the ECHR, and the UNCRPD, as well as national laws and institutional policies – mandate that restraint use be governed by strict safeguards, including valid informed consent, clear documentation, continuous monitoring, and external oversight. Embedding ethical decision-making models within institutional protocols, supported by legal regulations and professional guidelines (e.g., WHO, ANA, Joint Commission), is essential to ensure that restraint practices are ethically defensible, legally compliant, and aligned with a rights-based model of care. Ultimately, the responsible use, and preferably the progressive reduction, of PRs depends on cultivating a healthcare culture that consistently prioritizes ethical reasoning, legal accountability, and the protection of patient dignity.

Conflict of interest

The authors declare no conflict of interest.

Abbreviations

ANA	American Nurses Association
CRPD	Convention on the rights of persons with disabilities
ECHR	European Convention on Human Rights
JCAHO	Joint Commission on Accreditation of Healthcare Organizations
PR	Physical restraint
PRs	Physical restraints
UDHR	Universal Declaration of Human Rights
WHO	World Health Organization

Author details

Daisy Michelle Princeton[1*], Gülendam Hakverdioğlu Yönt[2] and Sezer Kisa[1]

1 Oslo Metropolitan University, Oslo, Norway

2 Izmir Tinaztepe University, Izmir, Türkiye

*Address all correspondence to: daisy.princeton@oslomet.no

References

[1] Gulpers MJM, et al. Belt restraint reduction in nursing homes: Design of a quasi-experimental study. BMC Geriatrics 2010;**10**:11

[2] Lee D-CA, et al. Prevalence and variability in use of physical and chemical restraints in residential aged care facilities: A systematic review and meta-analysis. International Journal of Nursing Studies. 2021;**117**:103856. DOI: 10.1016/j.ijnurstu.2020.103856

[3] Burry L, Rose L, Ricou B. Physical restraint: Time to let go. Intensive Care Medicine. 2018;**44**(8):1296–1298

[4] Karajeh A, Mrayyan M. Physical restraints: Ethical and legal argumentation. Frontiers of Nursing. 2025;**12**:195–199

[5] Zhou J, et al. Moral dilemmas regarding physical restraints in intensive care units: Understanding autonomy, beneficence, non-maleficence and justice in the use of physical restraints. Journal of Multidisciplinary Healthcare. 2024;**17**:1619–1627

[6] Hakverdioğlu Yönt G, Kisa S, Princeton DM. Physical restraint use in nursing homes-regional variances and ethical considerations: A scoping review of empirical studies. Healthcare (Basel). 2023;**11**(15):2204

[7] Scheepmans K, et al. Reducing physical restraints by older adults in home care: Development of an evidence-based guideline. BMC Geriatrics. 2020;**20**:169

[8] Delvalle R, et al. Mechanical restraint in nursing homes in Brazil: A cross-sectional study. Revista Brasileira de Enfermagem. 2020;**73** Suppl 3: e20190509

[9] Möhler R, Meyer G. Attitudes of nurses towards the use of physical restraints in geriatric care: A systematic review of qualitative and quantitative studies. International Journal of Nursing Studies. 2014;**51** (2):274–288

[10] Bleijlevens MH, et al. Physical restraints: Consensus of a research definition using a modified delphi technique. Journal of the American Geriatrics Society. 2016;**64**:2307–2310

[11] Goethals S, Dierckx de Casterlé B, Gastmans C. Nurses' ethical reasoning in cases of physical restraint in acute elderly care: A qualitative study. Medicine, Health Care and Philosophy. 2013;**16**(4):983–991

[12] Negroni AA. On the concept of restraint in psychiatry. The European Journal of Psychiatry. 2017;**31**(3): 99–104

[13] Gastmans C, Milisen K. Use of physical restraint in nursing homes: Clinical-ethical considerations. Journal of Medical Ethics. 2006;**32**(3):148–152

[14] Foebel AD, et al. Physical restraint and antipsychotic medication use among nursing home residents with dementia. Journal of the American Medical Directors Association 2016;**17**:184.e9–14

[15] Robins LM, et al. Definition and measurement of physical and chemical restraint in long-term care: A systematic review. International Journal of

Environmental Research and Public Health 2021;**18**:3639

[16] Bioethics., I.C.f. *The Bioethical Implications of Medical Restraints*. 2015. Available from: https://bioetica.governo.it/en/opinions/opinions-responses/the-bioethical-implications-of-medical-restraints/ [Accessed: 2025-September-17]

[17] Gunawardena R, Smithard DG. The attitudes towards the use of restraint and restrictive intervention amongst healthcare staff on acute medical and frailty wards-a brief literature review. Geriatrics (Basel). 2019;**4**(3):50

[18] Saarnio R, Isola A. Nursing staff perceptions of the use of physical restraint in institutional care of older people in Finland. Journal of Clinical Nursing. 2010;**19**(21-22):3197–3207

[19] Salehi Z, et al. Factors behind ethical dilemmas regarding physical restraint for critical care nurses. Nursing Ethics. 2020;**27**:598–608

[20] Cortinhal V, Correia A, Fernandes S. Nursing ethical decision making on adult physical restraint: A scoping review. International Journal of Environmental Research and Public Health. 2024;**21**:75

[21] Jang SG, et al. Is physical restraint unethical and illegal?: A qualitative analysis of Korean written judgments. BMC Nursing. 2024;**23**:94

[22] Sharifi A, et al. The principles of physical restraint use for hospitalized elderly people: An integrated literature review. Systematic Reviews. 2021;**10**:129

[23] Butterworth H, Wood L, Rowe S. Patients' and staff members' experiences of restrictive practices in acute mental health in-patient settings: Systematic review and thematic synthesis. BJPsych Open. 2022;**8**(6): e178

[24] Nations., U. *Universal Declaration of Human Rights. General Assembly Resolution 217 A (III) 10 December 1948*. Available from: https://www.nationsonline.org/oneworld/declaration_of_human_rights.htm [Accessed: September-14]

[25] Rights., E.C.o.H. *Convention for the Protection of Human Rights and Fundamental Freedoms*. 1950. Available from: https://www.echr.coe.int/documents/d/echr/Archives_1950_Convention_ENG [Accessed: September-14]

[26] Commission., E. *United Nations Convention on the Rights of Persons with Disabilities*. Available from: https://commission.europa.eu/strategy-and-policy/policies/justice-and-fundamental-rights/disability/united-nations-convention-rights-persons-disabilities_en [Accessed: 2025-September-17]

[27] Duffy RM, Kelly BD. Can the World Health Organisation's 'QualityRights' initiative help reduce coercive practices in psychiatry in Ireland?. Irish Journal of Psychological Medicine. 2023;**40**(2):114–117

[28] The Joint Commission. New and Revised Restraint and Seclusion Requirements for Behavioral Health Care and Human Services Organizations. Oakbrook Terrace, IL, USA: The Joint Commission; 2024

[29] Atee M, et al. Physical restraint in older people: An opinion from the early career network of the international psychogeriatric association.

International Psychogeriatrics. 2024;**36**:995–1006

[30] Association., A.N. *Reduction of Patient Restraint and Seclusion in Health Care Settings: Revised Position Statement*. 2012; Available from: https://www.nursingworld.org/globalassets/docs/ana/ethics/ps_reduction-of-patient-restraint-and-seclusion-in-health-care-settings.pdf [Accessed: 2025-September-17]

[31] Association., A.P. *Resource Document on Seclusion or Restraint*. 2022. Available from: https://www.psychiatry.org/getattachment/e9b21b26-c933-4794-a3c4-01ad427eed91/Resource-Document-Seclusion-Restraint.pdf [Accessed: 2025-September-14]

[32] Acevedo-Nuevo M, et al. Ethical and legal considerations and recommendations for action in the physical restraint use in critically ill patients. Enfermería Intensiva. 2025;**36**(2):100497

[33] Dworkin G. The Theory and Practice of Autonomy. Cambridge: Cambridge University Press; 1988

[34] Beauchamp T, Childress J. Principles of biomedical ethics: Marking its fortieth anniversary. The American Journal of Bioethics. 2019;**19**(11):9–12

[35] Bioethics. NCO. *Dementia: Ethical Issues – A Guide to the Report*. 2009, Nuffield Council on Bioethics: London

[36] Crutchfield P, et al. The conditions for ethical application of restraints. Chest. 2019;**155**:617–625

[37] Wong WK, Bressington DT. Nurses' attitudes towards the use of physical restraint in psychiatric care: A systematic review of qualitative and quantitative studies. Journal of Psychiatric and Mental Health Nursing. 2022;**29**(5):659–675

[38] te Boekhorst S, et al. Quality of life of nursing-home residents with dementia subject to surveillance technology versus physical restraints: An explorative study. International Journal of Geriatric Psychiatry. 2013;**28**:356–363

[39] Cautin RL, Lilienfeld SO. The Encyclopedia of Clinical Psychology, 5 Volume Set. Hoboken, New Jersey, USA: Wiley-Blackwell; 2015

[40] Wen X, et al. Application of Joanna Briggs Institute physical restraint standards to critical emergency department patients following CONSORT guidelines. Medicine. 2020;**99**:e23108

[41] Cusack P, et al. An integrative review exploring the physical and psychological harm inherent in using restraint in mental health inpatient settings. International Journal of Mental Health Nursing. 2018;**27**:1162– 1176

[42] Ye J, et al. Physical restraint in mental health nursing: A concept analysis. International Journal of Nursing Sciences. 2019;**6**:343–348

[43] Dauvergne JE, et al. Prevalence and risk factors of the use of physical restraint and impact of a decision support tool: A before-and-after study. Nursing in Critical Care. 2024;**29**:987–996

[44] de Casterlé BD, Goethals S, Gastmans C. Contextual influences on nurses' decision-making in cases of

physical restraint. Nursing Ethics. 2015;**22**(6):642–651

[45] Spennato U, et al. Prevalence, risk factors and outcomes associated with physical restraint in acute medical inpatients over 4 years-a retrospective cohort study. Geriatrics (Basel). 2023;**8**:15

[46] Sequeira H, Halstead S. The psychological effects on nursing staff of administering physical restraint in a secure psychiatric hospital:'When I go home, it's then that I think about it'. The British Journal of Forensic Practice. 2004;**6**(1):3–15

[47] Smithard D, Randhawa R. Physical Restraint in the Critical Care Unit: A Narrative Review. The New Bioethics. 2022;**28**(1):68–82

[48] Mohr WK. Restraints and the code of ethics: An uneasy fit. Archives of Psychiatric Nursing. 2010;**24**(1): 3–14

[49] Rights., A.C.f.E.a.H. *The Ethical Use of Restraints: Balancing Dual Nursing Duties of Patient Safety and Personal Safety. ANA Center for Ethics and Human Rights, Revised Position Statement*. 2020, Available from: https://www.nursingworld.org/globalassets/practiceandpolicy/nursing-excellence/ana-position-statements/nursing-practice/restraints-position-statement.pdf [Accessed: 2025-September-18]

[50] Fields LM, Calvert JD. Informed consent procedures with cognitively impaired patients: A review of ethics and best practices. Psychiatry and Clinical Neurosciences. 2015;**69**(8):462–471

[51] Seedsman T. Aging, informed consent and autonomy: Ethical issues and challenges surrounding research and long-term care. OBM Geriatrics. 2019;**3**:1–1

[52] Demir Zencirci A. Use of physical restraints in neurosurgery: Guide for a good practice. In: Signorelli F, editor. *Explicative Cases of Controversial Issues in Neurosurgery*., London, United Kingdom: InTech. 2012;(6):1573–81

[53] Øye C, Jacobsen FF. Informal use of restraint in nursing homes: A threat to human rights or necessary care to preserve residents' dignity?. Health: An Interdisciplinary Journal for the Social Study of Health, Illness and Medicine. 2020;**24**(2):187–202

[54] Hurlock-Chorostecki C, Kielb C. Knot-So-Fast: A learning plan to minimize patient restraint in critical care. Dynamics (Pembroke, Ontario). 2006;**17**(3):12–18

[55] Øye C, Jacobsen FF, Mekki TE. Do organisational constraints explain the use of restraint? A comparative ethnographic study from three nursing homes in Norway. Journal of Clinical Nursing. 2017;**26**(13-14): 1906–1916

[56] Gjerberg E, et al. How to avoid and prevent coercion in nursing homes. Nursing Ethics. 2013;**20**:632–644

[57] Zencirci Demir A. Attitudes, informed consent obtaining rates and feelings about physical restraint use among nurses. Turkiye Klinikleri Journal of Medical Sciences. 2009;**29**(6):1573–81

[58] Bazzano LA, Durant J, Brantley PR. A modern history of informed consent and the role of key information. Ochsner Journal. 2021;**21**(1):81–85

[59] Ng IK. Informed consent in clinical practice: Old problems, new challenges. Journal of the Royal College of Physicians of Edinburgh. 2024;**54** (2):153–158

[60] Thomann S, et al. Restraint use in the acute-care hospital setting: A cross-sectional multi-centre study. International Journal of Nursing Studies. 2021;**114**:103807. DOI: 10.1016/j.ijnurstu.2020.103807

[61] Cheung PP, Yam BM. Patient autonomy in physical restraint. Journal of Clinical Nursing. 2005;**14** Suppl 1: 34–40

[62] Wang J, et al. Effects and Implementation of A Minimized Physical Restraint Program for Older Adults in Nursing Homes: A Pilot Study. Vol. **10**, Front Public Health; 2022; 959016

[63] Brugnolli A, et al. The effectiveness of educational training or multicomponent programs to prevent the use of physical restraints in nursing home settings: A systematic review and meta-analysis of experimental studies. International Journal of Environmental Research and Public Health. 2020;**17**:6738

[64] Evans LK, Strumpf NE. Tying down the elderly. A review of the literature on physical restraint. Journal of the American Geriatrics Society. 1989;**37**(1):65–74

[65] Lai CK. Nurses using physical restraints: Are the accused also the victims? - A study using focus group interviews. BMC Nursing. 2007;**6**:5

[66] Bellenger EN, et al. Prevention of physical restraint use among nursing home residents in Australia: The top three recommendations from experts and stakeholders. International Journal of Older People Nursing. 2019;**14**:e12218

[67] Guttman R, Altman RD, Karlan MS. Report of the council on scientific affairs. Use of restraints for patients in nursing homes. Council on scientific affairs, American Medical Association. Archives of Family Medicine. 1999;**8**(2):101–105

[68] Moss RJ, Puma JL. The Ethics of Mechanical Restraints. The Hastings Center Report. 1991;**21**(1):22–25

[69] Woodward M. Physical restraint of older people: A study of Australian practices. Australasian Journal on Ageing. 1998;**17**(4):177–183

[70] Castle NG. Nursing homes with persistent deficiency citations for physical restraint use. Medical Care. 2002;**40**(10):868–878

[71] Heinze C, Dassen T, Grittner U. Use of physical restraints in nursing homes and hospitals and related factors: A cross-sectional study. Journal of Clinical Nursing. 2012;**21**(7-8):1033–1040

[72] McBrien B. Exercising restraint: Clinical, legal and ethical considerations for the patient with Alzheimer's disease. Accident and Emergency Nursing. 2007;**15**(2):94–100

[73] Frank C, Hodgetts G, Puxty J. Safety and efficacy of physical restraints for the elderly. Review of the Evidence. Canadian Family Physician. 1996;**42**:2402–2409

[74] Donato TAA, P.l., Silva LCP, Moura LVC, Santos AA, Souza LF. Physical restraint in patients in intensive care units: Exploratory - a descriptive study. Online Brazilian Journal of Nursing. 2017;**16**:83–93

[75] Heeren P, et al. Staffing levels and the use of physical restraints in nursing homes: A multicenter study. Journal of Gerontological Nursing. 2014;**40**:48–54

[76] Huizing AR, et al. Organisational determinants of the use of physical restraints: A multilevel approach. Social Science & Medicine. 2007;**65**:924–933

[77] Peisah C, Jessop T, Breen J. A missed opportunity to improve practice around the use of restraints and consent in residential aged care: Limitations of the quality of care amendment (minimising the use of restraints) principles 2019. Australasian Journal on Ageing. 2020;**39**(3):292–296

[78] Lejman E, et al. The ethics of coercive treatment of people with dementia. Nursing Ethics. 2013;**20**: 248–262

[79] Estévez-Guerra GJ, Fariña-López E, Penelo E. [Medical prescription and informed consent for the use of physical restraints in nursing homes in the Canary Islands (Spain)]. Gaceta Sanitaria. 2018;**32**(1):77–80

[80] Sokol DK. The “four quadrants” approach to clinical ethics case analysis; an application and review. Journal of Medical Ethics. 2008;**34**(7):513–516

[81] Toh HJ, et al. Jonsen’s four topics approach as a framework for clinical ethics consultation. Asian Bioethics Review. 2018;**10**:37–51

[82] Gulpers MJ, et al. Preventing belt restraint use in newly admitted residents in nursing homes: A quasi-experimental study. International Journal of Nursing Studies. 2012;**49**:1473–1479

[83] Hall H, Smithard DG. A principlist justification of physical restraint in the emergency department. The New Bioethics. 2021;**27**(2):176–184

[84] Huang HC, et al. Risk factors associated with physical restraints in residential aged care facilities: A community-based epidemiological survey in Taiwan. Journal of Advanced Nursing. 2014;**70**:130–143

[85] Retsas AP. Survey findings describing the use of physical restraints in nursing homes in Victoria, Australia. International Journal of Nursing Studies. 1998;**35**(3):184–191

Chapter 11

Ethical Implications of Parental Decision-Making for Serial Amnioinfusions in Congenital Renal Failure

Omri-David Soffer

Abstract

Fetal interventions, such as serial amnioinfusions, represent a paradigm shift in maternal-fetal medicine by offering potential survival for fetuses diagnosed with congenital renal failure, a condition previously deemed universally fatal. However, these interventions pose complex ethical dilemmas, particularly in parental decision-making, informed consent, medical uncertainty, quality-of-life considerations, and the allocation of healthcare resources. This chapter explores how healthcare providers can ethically support parental decision-making in cases of experimental fetal therapies. The analysis highlights the challenges of obtaining truly informed consent in high-stakes, emotionally charged situations where medical uncertainty plays a significant role. Additionally, the chapter examines the subjective nature of quality-of-life assessments and the ethical tensions surrounding the just distribution of healthcare resources, particularly regarding access to experimental interventions. While some argue that offering such therapies is an essential expression of parental autonomy and hope, others contend that doing so risks prolonging suffering and misallocating limited medical resources. A structured ethical framework balancing autonomy, beneficence, and justice is necessary to guide parental counseling and healthcare policy. By integrating shared decision-making models and transparent resource allocation policies, clinicians can support ethically sound, informed parental choices while promoting equity in access to fetal therapy. Future research should focus on improving long-term outcome data and refining ethical guidelines to ensure that these emerging medical interventions are both medically and ethically justifiable.

Keywords: fetal interventions, decision-making, amnioinfusions, parental autonomy, justice in healthcare

1. Introduction

Ruth and David sit silently in the exam room, the unclear ultrasound image still displayed on the screen. Their obstetrician, Dr. Joy, speaks carefully, her tone balancing empathy with clinical precision. "Your baby has no kidneys," she begins. "This means the kidneys cannot produce amniotic fluid, and without amniotic fluid, the lungs cannot develop properly. Without intervention, the prognosis is fatal."

Ruth becomes tearful as David grasps her hand. They have come to the hospital hoping for reassurance, but the news is devastating. Dr. Joy continues, "There is an experimental option – serial amnioinfusions. By restoring amniotic fluid, we can support the development of the lungs. It is not a cure, but it could give your baby a chance."

The word "chance" lingers in the room. Dr. Joy explains the procedure: weekly infusions into the amniotic sac, with risks of preterm labor and infection. If the baby survives birth, lifelong dialysis and a kidney transplant will likely be necessary. "It is a difficult decision," she says, "and I will be here to guide you every step of the way if you choose this path."

Over the next few weeks, Ruth and David grapple with the decision. Ruth is drawn to the hope of seeing their baby, whom they have already named Ethan, live beyond birth. "Even if it is just for a few years," she tells David, "he deserves a chance."

David hesitates, haunted by the potential suffering Ethan might endure. "Are we doing this for him or us?" he asks during one of their many late-night discussions.

In the clinic, Dr. Joy again walks them through the risks and benefits, emphasizing that there is no right or wrong choice – only what aligns with their values. Despite this support, Ruth and David feel the weight of the decision growing heavier with each passing day.

Finally, at 26 weeks of gestation, they chose to proceed. "We know it will not be easy," Ruth says, "but at least we will know we tried everything we could." As the first infusion begins, Ruth feels a flicker of hope, tempered by uncertainty.

This heart-wrenching dilemma is one that many parents of fetuses diagnosed with congenital renal failure now face due to emerging fetal interventions. Serial amnioinfusions represent a paradigm shift – transforming a once universally fatal condition into one with a possibility of survival. However, this possibility is not without ethical complications. How should healthcare providers ethically support parental decision-making in these cases?

This chapter explores how healthcare providers should ethically support parental decision-making regarding serial amnioinfusions in fetuses diagnosed with congenital renal failure. This question is critically important because it involves issues of informed consent, medical uncertainty, quality-of-life considerations, and distributive justice. Serial amnioinfusions challenge traditional notions of fetal viability and survival, compelling parents and clinicians to navigate complex ethical territory. While offering hope, this intervention introduces a range of complicated moral, emotional, and practical dilemmas that require thorough ethical analysis.

Additionally, the chapter addresses a growing ethical gap in maternal-fetal medicine. Advances in fetal therapy mean that conditions once deemed "lethal" are now associated with uncertain but nonzero survival outcomes. Unlike traditional interventions, serial amnioinfusions require parents to make a high-stakes decision based on limited evidence, with potential lifelong consequences for the child and family. The ability to frame and communicate these options in an ethical manner is crucial in ensuring that parents make informed, autonomous decisions that align with their values.

Lastly, the broader implications of fetal interventions extend beyond individual families. Who should have access to experimental treatments? How should healthcare systems strike a balance between hope and realism in their counseling? Should clinicians be obligated to offer fetal therapy, even when the long-term prognosis is unclear? Addressing these questions is necessary to guide future policy and clinical practice.

While this chapter aims to provide a robust ethical analysis of parental decision-making for serial amnioinfusions in fetuses diagnosed with congenital renal failure, it will not cover the clinical assessment of the procedure's medical efficacy. While discussions of survival rates, quality of life, and long-term outcomes are relevant to the ethical argument, this paper will not attempt to make a medical determination about whether serial amnioinfusions should be considered standard treatment. In addition, the legal implications of recommending or withholding experimental fetal therapy are beyond the scope of this paper. While informed consent laws and ethical guidelines will be discussed, legal frameworks such as wrongful life lawsuits or institutional liability for experimental procedures will not be analyzed in detail. Lastly, while religious and cultural beliefs may shape parental decision-making, this paper will not attempt to assess the moral permissibility of amnioinfusions through a theological or faith-based lens. Instead, the focus will be on bioethical principles applicable across diverse populations.

2. Medical uncertainty and parental decision-making

Parental decision-making in cases of experimental fetal interventions is particularly challenging due to medical uncertainty. Advances in maternal-fetal medicine have transformed the landscape of fetal interventions, presenting new possibilities for conditions that were once deemed universally fatal. One such condition is bilateral renal agenesis, in which a fetus develops without kidneys, leading to anhydramnios (low or absent amniotic fluid). In the past, this diagnosis meant certain death shortly after birth, as the lungs fail to develop without amniotic fluid, and the absence of kidney function makes postnatal survival nearly impossible [1].

However, experimental interventions such as serial amnioinfusions – a procedure in which amniotic fluid is repeatedly injected into the amniotic sac – have introduced the possibility of survival by promoting lung development before birth. Though these advances bring hope to families, they also introduce complex ethical dilemmas for parents and healthcare providers. Parents must make decisions about an intervention with uncertain long-term outcomes. Many infants who survive birth will still require lifelong dialysis and kidney transplants to survive, and their long-term quality of life remains unknown.

Medical uncertainty plays a critical role in shaping parental decision-making for serial amnioinfusions. Due to the experimental nature of this intervention, parents are faced with ambiguous information regarding potential outcomes, making truly informed consent challenging to achieve. While some infants born after serial amnioinfusions survive and go on to receive dialysis or kidney transplants, others may face severe complications, including preterm birth, respiratory distress, or early neonatal death [2].

Healthcare providers must navigate the delicate balance between instilling hope and ensuring that parents grasp the limitations of medical knowledge concerning this intervention. Studies show that parents facing medical uncertainty may struggle with decisional conflict, especially when the prognosis is ambiguous. One ethical challenge lies in reconciling the principle of autonomy with the provider's responsibility to prevent harm. Some ethicists contend that allowing parents to opt for serial amnioinfusions, despite limited evidence, could inadvertently expose neonates to prolonged suffering without guaranteeing a meaningful life expectancy [3].

On the other hand, medical uncertainty does not necessarily preclude ethical justification for offering experimental treatments. Some researchers suggest that, in cases where an intervention provides a chance for survival where none previously existed, denying access based solely on incomplete data could be seen as paternalistic and a violation of parental autonomy [4]. The most ethically sound approach involves a framework of shared decision-making in which healthcare providers transparently discuss known risks and unknowns while centering on parental values.

It is essential to acknowledge that, while uncertainty may increase the decisional burden, it does not automatically render a decision unethical. Rather than withholding the intervention due to a lack of conclusive data, healthcare providers should enhance their communication strategies. Providing parents with ethically grounded decision-making frameworks, multidisciplinary counseling, and access to other families who have undergone similar interventions could be instrumental in mitigating uncertainty while preserving parental autonomy.

Additionally, a shared decision-making model is recommended to address the challenges presented by medical uncertainty. Shared decision-making involves an ongoing dialogue between clinicians and parents, where medical professionals provide clear, evidence-based information while recognizing the limitations of current knowledge. This approach empowers parents to make informed choices that align with their values while ensuring that medical recommendations are ethically sound and balanced. Given the evolving nature of fetal therapies, transparent communication about risks, benefits, and uncertainties is crucial in promoting ethically responsible decision-making [5].

3. Informed consent

Informed consent is a cornerstone of ethical medical decision-making, but in cases of experimental fetal interventions, achieving truly informed consent is challenging. Parents must make emotionally charged decisions without precise data about the risks and benefits of the intervention [6].

Studies suggest that many parents struggle to fully understand complex medical information when they are in emotional distress [7]. Parents often rely on healthcare providers to guide their decision-making, which raises ethical concerns regarding potential provider bias. The way survival probabilities, risks, and burdens of treatment are framed significantly influences parental choices [8]. Some parents may feel pressured to pursue aggressive interventions if providers emphasize hope, while others may feel discouraged if providers focus on the likelihood of a poor prognosis.

Additionally, the distinction between directive and non-directive counseling is crucial. Some argue that physicians should actively guide parents toward what they believe to be in the child's best interest, while others maintain that true autonomy requires non-directive counseling [9, 10]. The most ethically sound approach likely lies between these extremes – a model in which providers offer structured guidance without unduly influencing the decision-making process.

I would argue that, while non-directive counseling protects autonomy, it may leave parents feeling abandoned when making a life-altering decision. A hybrid approach that offers expert medical guidance while respecting individual parental values is preferable. Implementing decision aids and structured counseling sessions, rather than one-time consent discussions, could bridge the gap between autonomy and physician guidance, ensuring truly informed decision-making. Parents must be given the full spectrum of information, including the uncertainties, medical burdens, and ethical considerations involved in each option. Nevertheless, clinicians should also help guide them through the process. Complete neutrality is neither realistic nor ethical when discussing high-stakes decisions with profound consequences. Instead of aiming for strict neutrality, providers should focus on clarity, transparency, and helping parents frame the decision in a way that aligns with their values.

Moreover, ensuring psychosocial support alongside medical counseling can improve the informed consent process. Decision-making frameworks should integrate palliative care teams and ethics consultations early in the process, allowing parents to explore what each option truly means for their child's future and their ability to provide long-term care.

Ultimately, informed consent in this context should not be viewed as a one-time event but as an ongoing, iterative process. Multidisciplinary counseling, involving neonatologists, ethicists, and social workers, can help ensure that parents receive balanced and comprehensive information.

4. Quality-of-life considerations

Assessing quality of life is central to ethical decision-making in neonatal and fetal care, yet it remains one of the most subjective and contested concepts in bioethics. In the context of serial amnioinfusion therapy for bilateral renal agenesis, discussions of quality of life are unavoidable. Infants who survive the intervention will almost certainly require intensive postnatal care, including respiratory support, dialysis, multiple surgeries, and eventual kidney transplantation. For many families, these realities raise the difficult question of whether the child's life – though biologically sustainable – will be meaningful or bearable, and for whom.

The principle of beneficence demands that healthcare providers act in ways that promote the well-being of patients. However, applying this principle in fetal medicine requires interpreting benefit from the perspective of a person who cannot yet speak for themselves and whose future quality of life is largely unknown. Critics of aggressive fetal interventions argue that survival at the cost of chronic pain, invasive treatments, and developmental limitations may represent a net harm rather than a benefit [11]. They question whether extending life without the possibility of a reasonably pain-free or autonomous existence serves the child's best interests. Furthermore, neonates who require long-term renal replacement therapy face frequent hospitalizations, painful procedures, risks of infection, and limited dietary and activity freedoms, placing them among the most medically complex pediatric populations [8].

Nonetheless, defining quality of life through a narrow medical lens risks marginalizing the lived experiences of children with disabilities and chronic illnesses. Disability rights advocates have long challenged assumptions that disability equates to diminished worth or suffering, emphasizing that many individuals with complex medical needs lead rich, meaningful lives – often because of, not despite, their unique experiences [8]. Parents, too, may perceive value in time spent with a child, however brief, framing meaning around love, connection, and legacy rather than functional independence or survival duration. This subjectivity underscores the ethical imperative to include families in nuanced, open-ended conversations about what constitutes an acceptable quality of life from their perspective, not just from a clinical standpoint.

Healthcare providers must, therefore, navigate a delicate balance. On one hand, they have an obligation to provide honest, evidence-based information about likely outcomes, including the burdens of care, potential suffering, and limitations on future autonomy. On the other hand, they must remain open to a range of parental values and avoid projecting their own quality-of-life judgments. Ethically, providers should not equate disability with suffering, nor presume that a medically complex child's life is inherently less worthy. Instead, they should help families explore what a meaningful life might look like within the boundaries of the likely medical trajectory.

Importantly, discussions about quality of life should extend beyond the individual child to encompass *family quality of life*, including caregiver burden, emotional resilience, and financial strain. Parents of children with end-stage renal disease face significant psychosocial challenges, including high rates of anxiety, depression, marital strain, and burnout. Siblings may also be affected by resource diversion and emotional distress [7]. Ethical counseling must therefore encompass the broader family system while avoiding the implication that a child's right to life is contingent upon the convenience or capacity of others.

To better inform these discussions, clinicians should consider drawing on the experiences of families who have navigated similar paths. Peer support networks, narrative medicine approaches, and family testimonials can help reframe abstract concepts like "quality of life" into more relatable terms. Hearing from parents of children on dialysis or with transplants can offer a richer, multidimensional view – one that acknowledges hardship but also highlights resilience, joy, and unexpected sources of meaning. These insights can guide prospective parents in deciding whether the future they are considering feels consistent with their hopes and values.

Another crucial consideration is the role of time. In some cases, families may pursue serial amnioinfusions not in expectation of long-term survival but in order to have a brief period of bonding – minutes, hours, or days – with their child outside the womb. In such cases, the goal is not necessarily to ensure a conventional notion of quality of life, but to experience a dignified introduction and farewell. These motivations are deeply personal and morally complex, but can be ethically valid, provided they are made with full understanding and intention. It is essential that clinicians explore and validate these narratives without defaulting to assumptions about futility or irrationality.

Ultimately, the ethical evaluation of quality of life in this context must embrace pluralism, humility, and transparency. Providers should foster environments where parents feel safe expressing their fears, hopes, and doubts, and where medical facts are presented alongside acknowledgment of their limits. A balanced, non-judgmental, and value-sensitive approach enables parents to define what constitutes a life worth living for their child, their family, and themselves. In doing so, the healthcare team honors not only the principle of autonomy but also the deeper ethical mandate to accompany families through uncertainty with compassion and moral clarity.

5. Justice and resource allocation

Justice in healthcare ethics demands equitable resource distribution, raising significant ethical concerns regarding the accessibility of experimental fetal interventions like serial amnioinfusions. These procedures require highly specialized maternal-fetal care and neonatal support, creating financial and systemic burdens that may not be justifiable in all cases [2].

Some ethicists argue that prioritizing resource allocation for interventions with uncertain long-term benefits diverts funding from neonates with more favorable prognoses. Neonatal and pediatric intensive care units already operate under resource constraints, and experimental fetal therapies place additional strain on healthcare systems. Hospitals must weigh the ethical justification of offering experimental treatments that may yield only marginal improvements in survival or quality of life against the need to support neonates who have a higher likelihood of survival and long-term well-being with proven interventions [12]. These concerns are particularly relevant in public healthcare systems, where resource allocation decisions have far-reaching implications for access to care across different patient populations. From a policy perspective, determining eligibility criteria for fetal interventions remains a pressing issue, particularly as emerging therapies continue to challenge traditional definitions of medical necessity and feasibility. Conversely, restricting access to serial amnioinfusions based on economic considerations alone risks reinforcing inequities in maternal-fetal healthcare. Critics contend that denying access due to cost-effectively discriminates against infants with disabilities and congenital anomalies [9]. A just healthcare system must strike a balance between individual rights to treatment and broader societal obligations.

I argue that the justice argument should extend beyond financial considerations to include broader systemic biases that affect maternal-fetal care. In many cases, access to experimental interventions is already stratified by socioeconomic status, with wealthier families having greater opportunities for experimental fetal therapies. Ethical guidelines for resource allocation must ensure that financial status does not become the primary determinant of access. Policymakers and healthcare institutions should establish equitable access policies that prioritize need over financial privilege, ensuring that justice considerations align with the ethical principles of beneficence and fairness [1].

6. Conclusion

The ethical support of parental decision-making for serial amnioinfusions requires a deliberate, structured, and compassionate approach that bridges the gap between medical innovation and moral responsibility. These cases sit at the crossroads of hope and uncertainty, demanding nuanced engagement from healthcare providers, ethicists, and policymakers alike.

First and foremost, medical uncertainty must be reframed not as an impediment but as a core feature of emerging fetal interventions that necessitate improved counseling strategies and shared decision-making models. Rather than deterring access, uncertainty should prompt more robust ethical dialogue, ensuring that parents are equipped with both clear information and empathetic guidance. Clinicians should be proactive in helping families navigate the emotional weight of these decisions, combining evidence-based medicine with narratives that contextualize survival data, potential complications, and long-term caregiving realities.

Moreover, this discourse underscores the necessity of institutional and policy-level engagement. Ethical considerations surrounding serial amnioinfusions are not confined to the bedside; they ripple outward into questions of distributive justice, equitable access, and systemic bias. Policymakers must recognize that limiting access to experimental fetal therapy based on cost or institutional capacity risks entrenching disparities in maternal-fetal care. Developing transparent eligibility criteria, investing in specialized centers of excellence, and creating national registries for outcome tracking could help ensure equitable and ethically defensible access.

The role of ethics consultation services is also paramount. Early integration of clinical ethicists, palliative care teams, and psychosocial support can reduce decisional conflict, foster clearer communication, and ensure that parental values remain central to the decision-making process. Institutions should embed these services within fetal care programs as a standard of practice, acknowledging the moral complexity inherent in experimental therapies.

Looking ahead, the ethical landscape of fetal interventions, like serial amnioinfusions, will evolve in tandem with advances in maternal-fetal medicine. Future research must prioritize longitudinal studies assessing neurodevelopmental outcomes, quality of life, and family burden to inform both counseling and policy. Such evidence will allow for dynamic ethical frameworks that adapt as our understanding deepens, ensuring that clinical practice remains grounded in compassion, justice, and respect for human dignity.

Ultimately, serial amnioinfusions force medicine to grapple with profound questions: What constitutes a life worth saving? How should hope be balanced against suffering? What obligations do we hold to future children and their families when our interventions fundamentally alter the trajectory of their lives? These questions cannot be answered solely by science; they demand interdisciplinary reflection and continuous ethical refinement.

At its core, this chapter calls for a vision of fetal medicine rooted not only in technical capability but also in humanity. Serial amnioinfusions are emblematic of a broader paradigm shift, where the boundaries between possibility and permissibility grow increasingly fluid. To navigate this terrain responsibly, we must embrace humility, prioritize transparency, and commit to ongoing dialogue that honors both parental autonomy and our collective ethical duties.

By anchoring parental decision-making within a framework that integrates beneficence, autonomy, and justice, we can move toward a model of care that not only saves lives but does so in a way that upholds the dignity and values of all involved. In doing so, we not only respond to the challenges of today but also lay the ethical foundation for the future of fetal medicine – one that is as principled as it is progressive.

Conflict of interest

The author declares no conflict of interest.

Thanks

I am thankful to my colleagues at Children's Nebraska and the University of Nebraska Medical Center, particularly those in the Fetal Care and Neonatal Intensive Care teams, for their collaboration and shared commitment to ethically grounded care. Their real-world experiences and ethical reflections have significantly informed the themes explored in this chapter.

Special thanks to the families. I have had the privilege of accompanying in the care of infants with congenital renal anomalies. Their strength, vulnerability, and decision-making in the face of uncertainty continue to inspire and challenge my ethical practice.

Author details

Omri-David Soffer
University of Nebraska Medical Center, Omaha, NE, United States

*Address all correspondence to: David.Soffer@unmc.edu

References

[1] Miller JL, Baschat AA, Rosner M, et al. Neonatal survival after serial amnioinfusions for bilateral renal agenesis: The renal anhydramnios fetal therapy trial. JAMA. 2023;**330** (21):2096–2105. DOI: 10.1001/jama.2023.21153.

[2] Soffer OD, Mauch TJ, Muff-Luett MA. Ethical concerns for amnioinfusions to treat early-onset anhydramnios. JAMA. 2023;**329** (22):1913–1914. DOI: 10.1001/jama.2023.6329.

[3] Chervenak FA, McCullough LB. Ethics in obstetrics and gynecology. An overview. European Journal of Obstetrics, Gynecology, and Reproductive Biology. 1997;**75**(1):91–94. DOI: 10.1016/s0301-2115(97)00192-9.

[4] Sundean LJ, McGrath JM. Ethical considerations in the neonatal intensive care unit. Newborn and Infant Nursing Reviews. 2013;**13**(3):117–120. DOI: 10.1053/j.nainr.2013.07.002.

[5] Lantos JD. Ethical problems in decision making in the neonatal ICU. The New England Journal of Medicine. 2018;**379**(19):1851–1860. DOI: 10.1056/NEJMra1801063.

[6] Butler CR, Wightman AG. Beyond autonomy: Ethics of decision-making about treatments for Kidney failure at the extremes of age. American Journal of Kidney Diseases. 2023;**82**(3):360–367. DOI: 10.1053/j.ajkd.2023.01.451.

[7] Gutman T, Hanson CS, Bernays S, Craig JC, Sinha A, Dart A, Eddy AA, et al. Child and parental perspectives on communication and decision-making in pediatric CKD: A focus group study. American Journal of Kidney Diseases. 2018;**72**(4):547–559. DOI: 10.1053/j.ajkd.2018.05.005.

[8] Wilkinson D, de Crespigny L, Xafis V. Ethical language and decision-making for prenatally diagnosed lethal malformations. Seminars in Fetal and Neonatal Medicine. 2014;**19**(5):306–311. DOI: 10.1016/j.siny.2014.08.007.

[9] Noble R, Rodeck CH. Ethical considerations of fetal therapy. Best Practice and Research: Clinical Obstetrics and Gynaecology. 2008;**22** (1):219–231. DOI: 10.1016/j.bpobgyn.2007.07.008.

[10] Minkoff H, Ecker J. Balancing risks: Making decisions for maternal treatment without data on fetal safety. American Journal of Obstetrics and Gynecology. 2021;**224**(5):479–483. DOI: 10.1016/j.ajog.2021.01.025.

[11] Rees L. Renal replacement therapies in neonates: Issues and ethics. Seminars in Fetal and Neonatal Medicine. 2017;**22**(2):104–108. DOI: 10.1016/j.siny.2016.11.001.

[12] Truog RD, Brock DW, Cook DJ, Danis M, Luce JM, Rubenfeld GD, Levy MM. Rationing in the intensive care unit. Critical Care Medicine. 2006;**34** (4):958–971. DOI: 10.1097/01.CCM.0000206116.10417.D9.

Chapter 12

Perspective Chapter: Economization/Commercialization in Medicine – Ethical Aspects

Franz Staudt

Abstract

Economization and commercialization have led to significant changes in the healthcare system in recent years, with severe repercussions for pediatric and adolescent medicine. As a result, the medical profession is being called into question, and the doctor-patient relationship is being seriously threatened. The following paper primarily describes the situation in the Federal Republic of Germany, with a particular focus on doctors and hospitals. The fundamentals of medical ethics, such as the four-principle model and the Geneva Pledge, are helpful for the ethical assessment of the resulting questions. The diagnosis-related groups (DRG), the profit-oriented financial investors and corporations, and the over-treatment for economic/commercial reasons are discussed. Bonuses for chief physicians, the COVID-19 pandemic, and their relation to ethics in medicine are mentioned. Medical-ethical and economic principles outlined here also apply to all those working in the healthcare sector. After all, the patient, or the human being, is at the center of the healthcare system.

Keywords: economization/commercialization, medical ethics, four-principle model, pediatrics, diagnosis-related groups, profit-orientation, bonuses, COVID-19 pandemic

1. Introduction

Economization and commercialization have led to significant changes in the healthcare system in recent years. This has had serious consequences for outpatient and inpatient care, with severe repercussions for pediatric and adolescent medicine [1]. This development is increasingly being criticized by doctors, nurses, and medical ethicists [2] As a result, the medical profession is being called into question, and the doctor-patient relationship is being seriously threatened. The following paper primarily describes the situation in the Federal Republic of Germany, with a particular focus on doctors and hospitals. However, the medical-ethical and economic principles outlined here also apply to all those working in the healthcare sector, as well as to administrators and investors. After all, the patient, or the human being, is at the center of the healthcare system [3].

2. The economic dimension of medicine today

The healthcare system in Germany has assumed a significant economic dimension. For 2017, the Federal Statistical Office (Destatis) [4] calculated an increase in healthcare spending of 4.9% compared to 2016, reaching €374.2 billion. From 2015 to 2016, spending had already increased by 3.8% to €356.5 billion, or €4,330 per inhabitant. This corresponded to 11.3% of gross domestic product (GDP). Healthcare spending in Germany has thus exceeded the €1 billion per day mark [5]. This is the highest figure in the EU [6]. Nevertheless, Germany ranks last among all 22 Western European nations in terms of life expectancy for German men, for example [7].

In 2022, healthcare spending in Germany rose again by 4.8%, or €22.6 billion, to €497.7 billion compared to the previous year. That amounted to 5,939 euros per inhabitant. According to the Federal Statistical Office (Destatis), healthcare spending accounted for 12.8% of GDP in 2022 [8].

2.1 Economization in the healthcare sector

Given the spiraling costs of healthcare, there is growing pressure to limit expenses. Health insurance companies, hospital operators, administrations, the Association of Statutory Health Insurance Physicians, and politicians are responding to this with enormous financial pressure on medical practice. This affects an area of public services where the primary concern should be the well-being of patients, not maximizing profits. However, the well-being of patients, that is, the protection of life and health, is and remains a fundamental right. It is considered the guiding principle in all medical ethical considerations regarding economization in the healthcare system.

Healthcare is a central part of social welfare, which is primarily concerned with the health and well-being of people. Given the high costs of healthcare, those responsible naturally have a high ethical obligation to use the available resources economically and sensibly, that is, sparingly and efficiently. Such appropriate "economization" must be clearly distinguished from irresponsible "commercialization" of the healthcare system, which pursues economic success or profit maximization as its primary value and places a higher value on this than on health or medically responsible care for patients.

Nevertheless, the terms economization and commercialization are often not distinguished as clearly as would be necessary for the discussion. Economization and commercialization differ in the following ways:

- economic efficiency, as opposed to commercialization, threatens the health, social, and ecological fabric of society [9];
- careful use of scarce resources, as opposed to purely market-based competition;
- increasing efficiency as opposed to increasing returns; and
- patient orientation, as opposed to profit or financial gain.

The former president of the Berlin Medical Association, Jonitz [10], emphasizes this distinction and makes it clear: "Under the current commercialization of the healthcare system, which is desired by politicians, there can be no functioning medical ethics." He also quotes Bert Brecht in this context: "First comes the food, then the morals – it's as simple as that" [11].

2.2 Fundamentals of medical ethics

In hardly any other profession is there such an ancient and demanding moral code as the Hippocratic Oath, the essence of which is represented by the four-principle model according to Beauchamp [12]. It includes:

- Respect for the autonomy of the patient (autonomy)
- Non-maleficence
- Beneficence
- Justice

The patient, as a person, is therefore at the center of all considerations for the common good, both in terms of their autonomy as an individual and in terms of justice within the framework of a solidarity-based community.

The modern implementation of the Hippocratic Oath is the Geneva Declaration, which was adopted by the General Assembly of the World Medical Association (WMA) in 1948. Unfortunately, however, many medical professionals are unaware that the resulting "Geneva Declaration" [13] forms the preamble to the professional code of conduct binding on all doctors within the state medical associations.

This declaration has been revised several times, most recently in 2017 [14], when patient autonomy was included in the pledge. This replaced the former patriarchal ethic of care with the concept of informed consent. This paradigm shift also has consequences for actions taken under economic considerations. Unfortunately, however, economics does not appear in either the Hippocratic Oath or the Geneva Declaration, but it is a matter of particular concern to the medical profession.

2.3 The necessity of economic and medically ethical action

The so-called magic square of health economics is a helpful approach to the question of how scarce resources can ultimately be distributed fairly [15]. The quality of care is reflected in the outcome. The performance or effectiveness of an institution and its economic efficiency are measured in terms of cost-effectiveness. This results in a close relationship with justice and the other medical-ethical principles mentioned above.

Economic thinking is a necessity, also in the interests of the healthcare system and thus of patients and contributors [16]. However, economics must not determine medical practice; rather, it should enable it! Doctors are constantly expected to think economically, but it is just as important that economists learn to think in terms of medical ethics [17].

However, doctors must not relinquish their primary responsibility to the administration, and the two areas are called upon to cooperate closely [18].

3. Consequences of unethical economization and commercialization

But what is the reality? In almost all areas of medical practice, the consequences of excessive economization and commercialization are evident:

Above all, the increasing privatization of what were originally public services based on solidarity has led to a massive increase in profit orientation, pushing medical ethics and necessity into the background [19]. Medical care has become considerably more bureaucratic for billing and liability reasons. This has resulted in an excessive system of regulations and controls that require detailed documentation.

However, this ties up a large part of working time. At the same time, qualities that cannot be measured but are of high ethical value, such as personal attention and care, have been devalued. For individual doctors, but also clinics, this results in burdens in the form of pressure from competition, rationing, budgets, and flat-rate payments, and ultimately an increase in financial risks, for example, in the form of recourse claims.

4. Diagnosis-related groups (DRG)

The German Health Structure Act of January 1, 1993 [20] replaced the previous system of daily nursing rates with retrospective reimbursement with a prospective flat-rate remuneration system based on DRGs. This system was essentially adopted from the Australian healthcare system but was introduced in an even more comprehensive form. As a result, politicians, the public sector, and health insurance companies shifted the financing risk to individual hospitals. This often had fatal consequences for hospitals providing basic care [18].

Unfortunately, the DRG system also leads to significant misguided incentives that harm patients [21]: First, there is "upcoding," that is, the exaggeration of diagnoses to generate higher revenues. Other examples of misguided incentives include revenue-driven premature discharges, known as "bloody discharges," restrictions on services within the flat rate, and care provided only on a minute-by-minute basis. Added to this is the so-called case splitting, that is, the division of complex cases into better-paid individual cases, or the provision of care exclusively based on the referral or main diagnosis instead of comprehensive treatment, and, unfortunately, also the performance of procedures that are not indicated for reasons of increased utilization and profitability.

A particular evil is the so-called departmental budgets. The individual departments of hospitals are subtly pressured by a business efficiency and competition logic [18], whereby the revenues from lucrative departments, such as orthopedics or cardiology, are compared with those of the generally weaker departments, in particular the pediatric clinics, which, in many cases, are loss-making. Accordingly, patients are categorized as either profitable or undesirable based on economic criteria. This is ethically unacceptable according to the principle of personal dignity.

Another unethical effect of the flat-rate payment is the manipulation of patient length of stay for billing reasons. Take "traumatic brain injury" as an example: If a patient is discharged after just one day, even though the minimum length of stay has not been reached, and does not stay in the hospital for two days, the hospital loses almost €500 per case. If this aspect is extrapolated over a year, the sums involved are considerable. A doctoral student at LMU Munich therefore came to the following recommendation in 2013: "Patients should not be discharged from the hospital after the first day or on the third or fourth day, but always on the second day of their stay" [22]. A prospective doctor who learns to think this way will probably focus first on profit and only then on the patient's well-being [23].

Another example is the birth weight-related revenues in neonatology: Their statistics show impressive jumps, for example, a doubling of revenues for premature babies above and below 1,000 grams. Considering the high costs of intensive care for premature babies, it is thought-provoking that the follow-up care for these children, who are often at risk of disability, has to be financed by donations because payment is based on the baby's weight category rather than the severity of the case.

The documented admission weights of premature babies are revealing and self-explanatory [24]. Before revenue-relevant jumps in birth weight, there is a dip, followed by a significant increase. Similar results can be obtained when looking at the duration of ventilation in neonatology, which is also of great importance for revenue. This suggests that the decision to discontinue ventilation is not always based solely on the well-being of the child.

A special chapter within the DRG system is the so-called minimum volumes. It is worth taking a look at the catalog of minimum volumes of procedures and services for the accreditation of hospitals, for example, for total knee replacement.

A survey shows that "economic reasons increase the willingness to manipulate volumes." Of 1,432 chief physicians, 39% agreed that economic conditions in their field had led to excessive numbers of procedures. Among orthopedists and trauma surgeons, the figure was around 50%, and in cardiology, as high as 61% [25].

Nevertheless, many initially assumed that the introduction of DRGs had been a success. They believed that the system had become part of everyday life and that the goals of the legislature had largely been achieved. The incentives to increase efficiency had worked [26].

However, Montgomery, former president of the German Medical Association (BÄK), qualifies this view: He believes that there is no alternative. "However, it is wrong to finance the system 100% through DRGs, as has been shown in Germany" [27].

4.1 DRGs and pediatrics

In the system of DRGs, hospitals are only paid for the treatments they perform. However, they are not remunerated for services that are provided but not used, which is particularly necessary in acute care or pediatric and adolescent medicine. It's like only paying the fire department when there's a fire. Many people only realized how absurd this form of financing was during the coronavirus pandemic.

In the DRG system, specific prices are assigned to treatment cases. Hospitals that treat many lucrative cases and have relatively low costs can thus gain a financial advantage. Others suffer losses, for example, because they have to spend more on staff. This has led to fewer and fewer staff being employed to care for more and more patients, and certain treatments being carried out only because they are particularly lucrative, even if they are not medically necessary [28]. This has also raised the question in the political arena as to whether DRGs make sense in pediatric medicine [29].

4.2 The Australian model

The German DRGs developed enormous momentum and had a significant impact on the hospital system. They were modeled on the Australian system but were introduced much more comprehensively and applied more generally [30]. In contrast, inpatient stays in none of the eight Australian states are reimbursed exclusively through flat rates; instead, billing is based on "historical budgets." The individual states differ in their billing modalities. In the states of Victoria and South Australia, approximately 60% of inpatient services are billed using DRGs. However, the remaining portion is excluded from the flat rates. This includes hospital outpatient services, specialized services such as human genetics and dialysis. In South Australia, complex cases, such as intensive care patients, are billed using a daily rate model. Furthermore, most pediatric centers in these two states are excluded from the flat-rate payments on the grounds that they are not adequately reflected in the DRG system.

There are considerable differences between the various states. In some cases, "historical budgets" are increasingly being used. The costs of the previous year are compared with the services provided, incorporated into the planning for the following year, and claimed as a budget increase accordingly.

The administrative burden has increased exponentially since the introduction of DRGs: DRG officers have been hired in every German hospital and are assisted by coding specialists. Medical controlling and the doctors employed in this field have become a separate department, albeit one that is part of the administration.

However, there is one significant difference compared to Australia: In the German system, coding is a medical task for which specialists or senior physicians are generally responsible and devote the necessary time. In Australia, analyzing data and coding patient diagnoses and therapies is a non-medical activity and is carried out by professional coders based on the files after the patients have been discharged. They comb through the files and enter the DRGs into the computer system based on the information in the files. These "clinical coders" have one year of training in medical terminology or are qualified as "medical health information management officers." This means that medical staff are fully available to care for patients. The lower labor costs for coders also save money.

In Australia, the public healthcare system covers most of the costs. Only part of the funding comes from DRGs, so there's no such thing as "the Australian system." However, the Australian government's policy is increasingly aimed at limiting public care. For example, healthcare funding was a significant issue in the last election in 2025.

4.3 DRGs in OECD countries

Increasingly, OECD countries are abandoning the DRG system [31]. The ten OECD countries in question (the USA, Canada (Ontario), Australia, Germany, France, England, Poland, Austria, Denmark, and Norway) have taken measures to reform the DRG system after it was shown that the financing system has a direct influence on the type of patient care. When activity is rewarded with revenue, it leads to an increase in the volume of services. An oversupply of care leads to a reduction in the quality of treatment.

Four trends were identified within the OECD countries studied for the reorganization of the DRG system. These include the introduction of fixed budgets, which are paid independently of the volume of services, and episode-based remuneration. Five of the ten countries have introduced flat-rate budgets. Norway, for example, combines both systems in equal parts. The USA has already experimented with several programs. These programs are particularly successful when the treatment pathway is clear and standardized.

In Germany, the Bundestag passed the Hospital Care Improvement Act (KHVVG) on October 17, 2024 [32]. The law is intended to fundamentally change the financing of inpatient care. Flat rates per case will be replaced by flat rates per case, largely independent of the services provided. This is intended to secure the existence of hospitals that are needed. At the same time, non-essential hospitals will be reduced or converted. The necessary hospitals in rural areas will be secured by means of surcharges. Hospitals are also to be relieved of bureaucracy and economic pressure.

5. Special features of pediatrics

The phenomenon of economization or commercialization affects almost all social subsystems to varying degrees. However, this is particularly problematic in areas that are not characterized by economically driven decision-making, such as childhood and, in particular, pediatrics. It is "caught between ethics and economics" [33] and is often seen as an unprofitable, "burdensome appendage" within a general hospital. With its well-known characteristics, such as the additional time and personnel required for patient care and the resulting significantly higher personnel costs compared to adult medicine, these facts are not adequately reflected in the current DRG system [33]. As a result, many children's hospitals have to operate at a loss.

This raises the question of whether children are entitled to particularly good healthcare for reasons of distributive justice for those most in need, and whether they should even be given preferential treatment. This is not only relevant in the medical field [34]. For example, pediatric professional associations have long been calling for a security surcharge for children's hospitals. Remarkably, the German Ethics Council [35] also addressed this issue in great detail in 2016 and recommended that the DRG system be adapted for pediatric and adolescent medicine or decoupled from the flat-rate payment system. However, these recommendations have largely been ignored to date.

Thirty years ago, the UN Convention on the Rights of the Child established the primacy of the best interests of the child [36]. Article 3, paragraph 1, covers "all measures that affect children," especially the right to "the highest attainable standard of health." This requirement applies worldwide, which raises the question of how limiting services for kids fits with the UN Convention on the Rights of the Child.

Since the provision of services in hospitals was primarily triggered by economic factors under the DRG system, hospitals with the possibility of increasing case numbers and focusing on technical services and homogeneous, high-revenue patient groups have benefited. These opportunities are less available to clinics for pediatric and adolescent medicine, for example. Pediatric medicine requires special, age-specific care for patients, that is, time spent on medical and nursing activities. The spectrum of individual diseases is also broader than in adult departments. In addition, fixed costs and standby costs are comparatively high.

6. Profit-oriented financial investors and corporations

The global financial system has led to enormous amounts of money seeking profitable investments, especially in industrialized countries. High returns are usually the primary goal of profit-oriented financial investors and corporations, which are buying up more and more clinics and medical practices. As a result, clinics operated by large corporations or private healthcare providers are focusing on specialties that are both economically profitable and in demand, such as surgery and orthopedics, since elective (planned) surgical procedures, such as orthopedic surgery for degenerative diseases like osteoarthritis (hip and knee replacements) or injuries, are often profitable. Some privatized hospitals now only offer services that generate profits due to the flat-rate payment system. This "cherry-picking" means that other patients are referred to public hospitals, placing an additional burden on them. However, the high level of privatization and the creeping industrialization of the healthcare system are jeopardizing medical care [37].

For example, the expected returns of some hospital groups, up to 15%, are ethically questionable, especially if they are not primarily used for reinvestment but to maximize shareholder profits [16]. It is difficult to accept that a group with 110 clinics in Germany reports hundreds of millions in profits every year [43]. However, the desired return can hardly be achieved through increased efficiency alone. Personnel costs, especially in pediatrics, are known to account for the largest share of expenditures, so it stands to reason that savings will be made primarily in personnel, who will then be overworked, which can be particularly fatal in hospitals with acute care.

The Association of Scientific Medical Societies (AWMF) is, therefore, calling for privately-run hospitals to be operated exclusively as non-profit enterprises [38]. The Marburger Bund (German doctors' association) similarly complains that hospitals and medical practices must not be allowed to become objects of speculation and profit-making. Dr. Broß, a former judge at the Federal Constitutional Court, even takes the view that profit orientation in the hospital sector is unconstitutional [39].

There are calls for a move away from profit maximization [40]. Instead of putting patients' well-being at risk for the sake of profits, there are calls for evidence-based medicine through better integration of medical and clinical experience on the one hand, and the best possible use of medical research knowledge on the other [41].

7. Over-treatment for economic/commercial reasons

In Germany, it is not only the threat of undersupply that is causing problems, especially for patients in rural areas, but also over-treatment for economic or, more precisely, commercial reasons. In a statement by the Central Ethics Commission of the BÄK, it is stated that medically unindicated measures are carried out for "economic" reasons in order to maximize profits [42].

The risk of overtreatment is greatest at the end of life. With the attempt to prolong human life "at any cost," that is, for commercial reasons, overtreatment at the end of life becomes a paradox in the healthcare system [43].

The German Society for Internal Medicine (DGIM) has launched an initiative called "Klug entscheiden" (decide wisely) [44], which can provide important guidance in this area. It was inspired by the "Choosing Wisely" program launched by the American Board of Internal Medicine (ABIM) in 2012. The concept of "targeted omission" plays a special role in this context.

The BÄK and the WMA participated in the Vatican's Pontifical Academy "Pro-Vita" in 2017 on this topic [45]. Pope Francis referred to a speech by Pope Pius XII on the subject of "accepting death." He called for the prudent use of maximum therapy at the end of life and explicitly mentioned the withdrawal of therapy, or rather the "change of treatment goal," as a possible option in hopeless situations. In such cases, it is not a question of bringing about death but of accepting that it cannot be prevented and refraining from subjecting the patient to unethical – because pointless – treatment shortly before death for commercial reasons. This is where living wills, advance directives, and palliative care have a special place. The goal of palliative medicine is not to prolong life at all costs but to make the last days of life easier, for example, through pain relief, intensive care, and spiritual care, and to make them as livable as possible.

8. Limits of economization and commercialization

"Doctors and nurses experience in their everyday work that they can either act in the interests of economic interests (those of their employer or their own) or in the interests of their patients, and this puts them in a conflict of interest" [25]. The pressure of economic incentive systems creates a risk of calling into question the primacy of medical ethics and, thus, the freedom of doctors to make decisions and choose treatments [16].

Commercialized medicine does not cut out the superfluous but rather cuts into the core of its identity [18]. Humanity and care are lost. Quantity takes precedence over quality, while the patient becomes part of a "medical business," and the relationship of trust between doctor and patient [46] falls by the wayside. Although this relationship of trust is difficult to measure, it is an essential factor in healing. It is therefore not only ethically important but ultimately also economically significant.

Due to the intensification of work processes, consultations with patients can increasingly only take place after regular working hours. For doctors, this leads to overload and demotivation. "However, the medical profession must not be destroyed by pure economization. Otherwise, the dream job of being a doctor will become a nightmare" [27]. Prospective doctors are asking themselves whether they want to become doctors under these conditions.

It is also a principle that doctors must not accept instructions from non-doctors regarding their medical decisions. "But the opposite is now a daily reality." Many doctors, especially those in management positions, no longer even notice how much the system has reprogrammed them. They give in to economic pressure and "step by step make the foreign logic of economics their own" [18]. Many believe that they must act in this way for the good of their hospital. We therefore need a new self-image and a "new self-confidence!" [17]

9. Hospital reform in Germany through the Hospital Remuneration Act (KHEntgG)

In 2024, politicians responded to widespread criticism of the DRG system. The current hospital reform, or rather the reform of the KHEntgG (Krankenhausentgeltgesetz/Hospital Remuneration Act) through the KHVVG (Krankenhausversorgungsverbesserungsgesetz/Hospital Care Improvement Act) of December 11, 2024, essentially provides for changing the remuneration system with flat rates for treatment cases to significantly improve the quality of hospital treatment and ensure comprehensive care [47].

Hospitals are to be relieved of the economic pressure to take on more and more cases and, in some instances, to perform procedures for which they do not possess a high level of expertise. Instead, they are to receive a significant proportion of their remuneration simply for providing staff, technology, emergency rooms, and other services. Rather than the DRG's flat rates that have been the norm up to now, there will be provision budgets in the future.

Funding by health insurance companies will be based on more precisely defined service groups for hospitals, which will ensure uniform quality standards in terms of equipment, staffing, and treatment experience. Five additional, technically necessary service groups will be added: Infectious diseases, emergency medicine, specialized traumatology, specialized pediatric and adolescent medicine, and specialized pediatric and adolescent surgery.

Additional financial resources amounting to €300 million have been made available for the care of children and adolescents in 2023 and 2024. From 2027 onwards, these will be financed through increased reserve assessment ratios for pediatric service groups. For 2025 and 2026, a surcharge for the treatment of pediatric cases is to be introduced for hospitals and special facilities in order to secure funding for additional support during these years as well [48].

Furthermore, the hospital network is to be classified into levels, ranging from basic care close to home to standard and specialized care to maximum care, for example, in university hospitals. Concrete implementation in local hospitals is then to begin gradually. However, it is to be expected that more hospitals will go bankrupt before the reform takes effect.

10. Bonuses for chief physicians

Hospital operators repeatedly attempt to agree on bonuses in contracts with senior physicians for the achievement of contractually agreed targets. The BÄK and the Association of Senior Hospital Physicians in Germany have made a clear statement on this issue [49]. If bonuses are linked to medically meaningful, patient-oriented goals (e.g., quality of treatment, patient satisfaction, further training of staff) and thus create incentives for better care, they may be permitted. Since chief physicians also have management responsibilities (e.g., budget and personnel management), bonuses can appropriately reward their role as medical leaders.

There is a risk that these bonuses will push ethical principles into the background. Bonuses are ethically problematic in any case if they are linked to case numbers, and a chief physician receives additional remuneration for each operation or inpatient admission, or even for a certain number of premature babies below a certain birth weight.

This can lead to an increased risk for patients and the misuse of resources for medically unnecessary treatments, and when economic interests prevail, the medical ethos is undermined.

11. COVID-19 pandemic

The COVID-19 pandemic has raised a variety of ethical questions and challenges. It has exacerbated existing inequalities in access to health services. Problems arose regarding the equitable distribution of resources, such as vaccines and medical care. Of central importance was how to protect risk groups (older people, people with pre-existing conditions) and how to ensure that children, for example, were not disadvantaged [50]. The ethical question arose as to how these groups could be prioritized without discriminating against others.

The debate on the introduction of compulsory vaccination raises ethical questions, particularly with regard to individual freedom and the right to self-determination versus the protection of public health [51]. The equitable distribution of vaccines, both within countries and internationally, is also a key ethical issue.

Measures to contain the pandemic, such as lockdowns and restrictions on assembly, have led to debates about individual freedoms. This has also raised the question of the proportionality [52] of the measures. The use of technologies to track infections has come into conflict with issues of data protection and personal freedom.

In times of healthcare system overload, hospitals have had to make difficult decisions about the allocation of resources (e.g., ventilators and intensive care beds). This so-called triage has raised questions about the criteria that should be used to make such decisions [53].

The urgency of vaccine development has prompted consideration of the ethics of clinical trials, particularly regarding participant consent, speed of introduction, and transparency of research [53].

The psychological impact of lockdowns and social isolation has been significant. This has raised questions about the ethical responsibility to protect the mental health of those affected [54].

The pandemic has increased the need for psychotherapy, especially for children. This raises questions about the availability, accessibility, and financing of such measures. Discussing these issues is crucial in order to learn from the results and mistakes, and to find fair and sustainable responses to the challenges that may arise from pandemics similar to the COVID-19 pandemic.

In the first months of the COVID-19 pandemic, significant financial resources were spent on masks, tests, and other protective measures. Speed was of the essence, but there was a lack of relevant experience [55].

Many people and experts considered the spending necessary. The goal was to protect healthcare systems and contain the spread of the virus. Investments in masks, tests, and vaccines have helped to better control the pandemic and reduce severe cases of the disease. On the other hand, the high costs are being critically questioned, especially with regard to efficiency, appropriateness (proportionality), and the long-term financial consequences. Many countries are rethinking and improving their existing strategies to better cope with future pandemics.

During the COVID-19 pandemic, there were cases of fraud and self-interest, particularly in connection with the purchase of masks [54]. Some retailers or suppliers charged excessive prices or sold counterfeit products. Even ministers came under suspicion of acting out of self-interest [56].

A crisis such as the COVID-19 pandemic drives politicians to act. Government measures to control and direct people seem justified on the grounds of subsidiarity and the common good. Hard-won democratic rights have been restricted. In Hungary and Poland, for example, this has been used as an opportunity to consolidate authoritarian rule. If we are aware of this and expect it to happen, we will defend ourselves more effectively and avoid falling into a state of shock [57].

12. Resistance to the commercialization of medicine

For several years now, resistance among doctors and patients to the commercialization of medicine has been growing. Our Swiss colleagues at the "Stiftung Dialog Ethik" (Ethics Dialog Foundation) have therefore drawn up a "new medical oath" [58], in which they promise, among other things: "I practice medicine with a sense of proportion and do not recommend or take any measures that are not medically indicated." They also vow: "I will not exploit my patients for career or other purposes."

Similarly, the German Society for Internal Medicine has formulated a "Clinic Codex" under the title "Medicine before Economics." [59] This code has since been renamed the "Physicians' Code," presumably to include colleagues in private practice. The German Society for Pediatrics and Adolescent Medicine supports this initiative by internists. The Marburger Bund also adopted a remarkable position paper on this subject in September last year. In the meantime, around 250 associations and doctors have issued an appeal to politicians and society, which has also been reported on in detail [60].

The Bavarian State Medical Association (BLÄK) generally recommends that the topic of ethics be more firmly anchored in further training and taken into account in practice. It demands that "medical ethics must be a topic of daily discussion" [61].

13. Review and outlook

The philosopher Immanuel Kant summed up the issue in the "purposive formula" of his categorical imperative: "Act so that you treat humanity, whether in your own person or the person of any other, always at the same time as an end, never merely as a means" [62]. This implies that the well-being of the patient should be the purpose of medical practice, but that the patient must never be abused as a means to an end, such as financial gain or career advancement.

The ancient maxim of ethics, the so-called "golden rule" [63], expresses the same idea in simpler words: "Do unto others as you would have them do unto you." The well-known saying puts it another way: "For pediatricians, this may become even clearer if we expand the sentence to say: What you do not want to be done to yourself, your child, or your grandchild, do not do to anyone else."

Finally, the Golden Rule should be supplemented [64] by the Platonic cardinal virtues of prudence, courage, wisdom, and justice [65]. Physicians should have the courage to act accordingly and find the right balance with prudence.

14. Conclusion

Germany spends over €1 billion per day on health (12.8% of GDP). This is the highest figure in the EU (€5,939 per capita per year) – but the return on this investment is insufficient. The distinction between necessary economization and unacceptable commercialization illustrates the problem. The four-principles approach to healthcare ethics (Beauchamp and Childress) is particularly relevant to economic issues in medicine.

Children occupy a special position in the medical ethics debate on the distribution of health resources, and this must be taken into account more strongly. The DRG system needs fundamental reform. It leads to profit orientation, medically and ethically wrong incentives, staff overload, and misuse of available resources. It is wrong to finance the healthcare system 100% through this system. It remains to be seen whether the hospital reform and the current reform of the Hospital Remuneration Act (KHEntgG) will succeed in providing a better solution in practice in Germany.

The economy should enable medical treatment, but it must not determine it. Doctors should think and act ethically and economically. However, it is just as important that economists and administrators learn to think and act according to medical ethics. Profit-oriented financial investors and corporations are jeopardizing adequate medical care, the relationship of trust between doctors and patients, and the reputation of doctors and the healthcare system itself through commercialization and the creeping industrialization of healthcare. Over-treatment at the end of life becomes a paradox when attempts are made to prolong human life for economic or even commercial reasons. Commercially motivated underprovision is equally reprehensible. Many doctors are bowing to economic pressure and, step by step, are adopting the logic of commercialization, which is alien to them, as their own. However, more and more doctors are suffering from the violation of their ethical obligations by their medical ethics. Bonuses for chief physicians are, therefore, questionable if they result in economic interests taking precedence and thus undermine the medical ethos.

The COVID-19 pandemic has raised many new ethical questions. It is medically ethical and economically necessary to learn the essential lessons for the future from the experiences and mistakes made. Resistance to the commercialization of medicine is growing, for example, through the "Dialog Ethik" foundation, the "Ärztecodex" (Physicians' Code of Conduct), which is already supported by 30 organizations, the position paper of the Marburger Bund, and the doctors' appeal against the dictates of economics in our hospitals, published by around 250 professional societies, associations, federations, and individual doctors. In this way, doctors are critically reflecting on the effects of economization and commercialization in their personal field of work and are looking for ways to make medically and ethically responsible decisions for their patients in their everyday work, while also using scarce resources in an economically responsible manner.

Author details

Franz Staudt
Former Medical Director of the Kinderklinik Dritter Orden, Passau, Germany

*Address all correspondence to: franz.staudt@t-online.de

References

[1] Staudt F. Ökonomie in der Medizin – Ethische Aspekte [Economics in medicine – Ethical aspects]. Monatsschrift Kinderheilkunde. 2020;**168**:828–833

[2] Heubel F, ed. Professionslogik Im Krankenhaus – Heilberufe Und Die Falsche Ökonomisierung, [Professional Logic in Hospitals - Healthcare Professions and the False Economization]. Frankfurt am Main: Humanities Online; 2015

[3] Second Vatican Council. Pastoral Constitution: Gaudium et spes on the Church in the Modern World, 25. The Mutual Dependence of the Human Person and Human Society. 1965. https://www.vatican.va/archive/hist_councils/ii_vatican_council/documents/vat-ii_const_19651207_gaudium-et-spes_en.html [Accessed: 2025-October-08]

[4] Statistisches Bundesamt (Federal Statistical Office). Gesundheitsausgaben pro Tag überschreiten Milliardengrenze [Daily healthcare expenditure exceeds billion mark]. 2018; https://www.destatis.de/DE/Presse/Pressemitteilungen/2018/02/PD18_050_23611.html [Accessed: 2025-October-08]

[5] Thelen P. Tägliche Gesundheitsausgaben knacken die Milliarden-Marke [Daily healthcare expenditure breaks the billion mark]. Handelsblatt. 2018

[6] Ärzteblatt.de. EU-Kommissar moniert „Überversorgung“ im deutschen Gesundheitswesen[EU Commissioner criticises “overprovision” in German healthcare system]. 2018. www.aerzteblatt.de/nachrichten/98804/EU-Kommissar-moniert-Ueberversorgung-im-deutschen-Gesundheitswesen [Accessed: 2025-October-08]

[7] Woratschka R. Europaweiter Vergleich: Warum haben Deutsche so eine geringe Lebenserwartung? [Europe-wide comparison: Why do Germans have such a low life expectancy?]. DER Tagesspiegel. November 21, 2018, https://www.tagesspiegel.de/politik/warum-haben-deutsche-so-eine-geringe-lebenserwartung-4011370.html [Accessed: 2025-October-08]

[8] Statistisches Bundesamt [Federal Statistical Office]. Gesundheitsausgaben im Jahr 2022 auf knapp 500 Milliarden Euro gestiegen [Healthcare spending to rise to just under €500 billion in 2022] https://www.presseportal.de/pm/32102/5765285 [Accessed: 2025-October-08]

[9] Ebner A. Theorie der Vermarktlichung: Ein institutionalistischer Ansatz [Theory of Marketization: An Institutionalist Approach]. In: Bögenhold D, ed. Soziologie Des Wirtschaftlichen. Wiesbaden: Springer VS; 2013. DOI: 10.1007/978-3-658-03545-7_4

[10] Jonitz G. Eid des Hippokrates – Ethisch unmöglich [Hippocratic Oath – Ethically Impossible], Frankfurter Rundschau. 2019-January-07. https://www.fr.de/ratgeber/gesundheit/ethisch-unmoeglich-11041734.html [Accessed: 2025-June-02]

[11] Ohl L. “Erst kommt das Fressen, dann die Moral”: Die Bedeutung des Sprichworts [“First Comes Food, Then

Morality": The Meaning of the Proverb]; 2025, https://praxistipps.focus.de/erst-kommt-das-fressen-dann-die-moral-die-bedeutung-des-sprichworts_184652 [Accessed: 2025-October-08]

[12] Beauchamp TL, Childress JF. Principles of Biomedical Ethics. 6th ed. Oxford: Oxford University Press; 2008

[13] Bundesärztekammer [German Medical Association]. (Muster-) Berufsordnung für die in Deutschland tätigen Ärztinnen und Ärzte, [(Model)–professional code for Physicians in Germany].2024. file:///C:/Users/user01/Downloads/_Bek_BAEK_Musterberufsordnung-AE1.pdf [Accessed: 2025-June-5]

[14] Parsa-Parsi R, Wiesing U. Weltärztebund: Revision des ärztlichen Gelöbnisses [World Medical Association. Revision of the Medical Oath]. DtschArztebl. 2017;**114**:44

[15] van der Beek K. Gesundheitsökonomik – Einführung [Health Economics – Introduction]. Munich: Oldenbourg Verlag; 2019

[16] Jörg J. Berufsethos Kontra Ökonomie [Professional Ethics versus Economic]. Berlin Heidelberg: Springer-Verlag; 2015. 7–21 p

[17] Hibbeler B. Ökonomisierung der Medizin: Die Grenzen des Marktes [The Economization of medicine: The limits of the market]. DtschArztebl. 2013;**110**:23–24

[18] Maio G. Geschäftsmodell Gesundheit [The Business Model of Health]. 2nd ed. Berlin: Suhrkamp Verlag; 2016

[19] Montgomery FU. Geleitwort: Ökonomisierung der Medizin: Den Patienten heilen und gleichzeitig den Kunden zufriedenstellen [Foreword: The economization of medicine: Healing patients while satisfying customers]. In: von Eiff W, ed. Ethik Und Ökonomie in der Medizin [Ethics and Economics in Medicine], Heidelberg: Medhochzwei Verlag GmbH. 2014

[20] Bundesministerium der Justiz (Federal Ministry of Justice). Gesetz zur Sicherung und Strukturverbesserung der gesetzlichen Krankenversicherung (Gesundheitsstrukturgesetz) [Law on the Security and Structural Improvement of Statutory Health Insurance (Health Structure Act)], 1992; www.gesetze-im-internet.de/gsg/BJNR022669992.html [Accessed: 2025-October-08]

[21] Roeder N, Hensen P, Franz D. Ed. Gesundheitsökonomie, Gesundheitssystem Und Öffentliche Gesundheitspflege [Health Economics, Healthcare System, and Public Health Care]. Köln: Deutscher Ärzte-Verlag; 2014

[22] Gebhardt Ph B. Kosten-Nutzenanalyse in der SHT (Schädel-Hirn-Trauma) – Diagnostik, [Cost-benefit Analysis in TBI (Traumatic Brain Injury) Diagnostics], dissertation, LMU Munich. Faculty of Medicine; 2013. Available at: https://edoc.ub.uni-muenchen.de/15691/ [Accessed: 2025-October-08]

[23] Haas NA. Themen der Zeit, Fallpauschalen: Die australische Realität [Topics of the Day, Flat-Rate Fees – The Australian Reality]. DtschArztebl. 2014;**111**(45)

[24] Abler SC. Vergleich der VLBW-Aufnahmegewichte in Sämtlichen NRW-Neonatologien Prä-Und post-DRG-Implementierung, [Comparison

of VLBW Admission Weights in All Neonatal Units in North Rhine-Westphalia before and after DRG Implementation], [dissertation, University of Duesseldorf], 2012

[25] Flintrop J. Krankenhäuser zwischen Medizin und Ökonomie: Die Suche nach dem richtigen Maß [Hospitals between medicine and economics: The search for the right balance]. DtschArztebl. 2014;**111** (45):1929

[26] Beivers A, Emde A. DRG-Einführung in Deutschland: Anspruch, Wirklichkeit und Anpassungsbedarf aus gesundheitsökonomischer Sicht. [Introduction of DRGs in Germany: Aspirations, reality, and the need for adjustment from a health economics perspective1]. In: Klauber J, Geraedts M, Friedrich J, Wasem J, Beivers A, eds. Krankenhaus-Report 2020 [Hospital Report 2020]. Berlin, Heidelberg: Springer; 2020. DOI: 10.1007/978-3-662-60487-8_1

[27] Hoppe J. quoted in Osterloh F. Patientenversorgung unter Druck - Gegen die Kommerzialisierung, [Patient care under pressure – Against commercialization]. DtschArztebl. 2018;**115**:48

[28] Knight B. Germany begins major reform of its hospital sector. 2024. https://www.dw.com/en/germany-begins-major-reform-of-its-hospital-sector/a-69236520 [Accessed: 2025-June-2]

[29] Rodeck B, Lutterbüse N, Krägeloh-Mann I. Diagnosis Related Groups in der Pädiatrie – Segen oder Unsinn? [Diagnosis Related Groups in Pediatrics – Blessing or Nonsense?]. Monatsschrift Kinderheilkunde. 2021;**169**:520–526

[30] Rochell B. Eingesetzte DRG-Varianten in Europa, Australien und USA. [DRG variants used in Europe, Australia, and the USA]. In C WD, D MM, W KE, eds. DRG's in Orthopädie Und Unfallchirurgie [Durgs in Orthopedics and Trauma Surgery]. Berlin, Heidelberg: Springer; 2004. DOI: 10.1007/978-3-642-18588-5_23

[31] Milstein R, Schreyögg J. The end of an era? Activity-based funding based on diagnosis-related groups: A review of payment reforms in the inpatient sector in 10 high-income countries. Health Policy. 2024;141,1–8

[32] Bundesministerium für Gesundheit [German Federal Ministry of Health]. Bundestag beschließt Krankenhausreform [Bundestag adopts hospital reform]. October-07-2024. www.bundesgesundheitsministerium.de/presse/pressemitteilungen/bundestag-beschliesst-krankenhausreform-pm-17-10-2024.html [Accessed: 2025-July-28]

[33] Weyersberg A, Roth B, Woopen C. Pädiatrie: Folgen der Ökonomisierung. [Pediatrics: Consequences of economization]. DtschArztebl. 2018;**115** (9)

[34] Hoburg R. Theologie der Helfenden Berufe [Theology of the Helping Professions]. Stuttgart: Verlag W. Kohlhammer; 2008. p. 66

[35] Deutscher Ethikrat [German Ethics Council] Patientenwohl als ethischer Maßstab für das Krankenhaus [Patient welfare as an ethical standard for hospitals]. 2016; www.ethikrat.org/fileadmin/Publikationen/Stellungnahmen/deutsch/stellungnahme-patientenwohl-als-ethischer-massstab-fuer-das-krankenhaus.pdf [Accessed: 2025-October-25]

[36] Straßburg M, Zimmer K-P. Versorgung von Kindern und

Jugendlichen: Warum die Kinderrechte in das Grundgesetz gehören [Care for children and adolescents: Why children's rights belong in the Basic Law]. DtschArztebl. 2018;**115**:46

[37] Bund M. Die negativen Folgen der Ökonomisierung der Gesundheitsversorgung [The negative consequences of the economization of healthcare] 2018; www.marburger-bund.de/nrw-rlp/meldungen/die-negativen-folgen-der-oekonomisierung-der-gesundheitsversorgung [Accessed: 2025-October-08]

[38] AWMF. Medizin und Ökonomie - Maßnahmen für eine wisssenschaftlich begründete, patientenzentrierte und ressourcenbewußte Versorgung [Medicine and economics – Measures for scientifically based, patient-centered, and resource-conscious care] 2018; www.awmf.org/fileadmin/userupload/Stellungnahmen/MedizinischeVersorgung/Medizinund-Ökonomie–AWMF_StrategiepapierV1.0mitLit.pdf [Accessed: 2025-October-08]

[39] Broß S Das Krankenhaus – Ein kommerzieller Wirtschaftsbetrieb? [The hospital – A commercial enterprise?]. 17th Federal Congress of the Federal Association of German Pathologists. Berlin, 2017-September 23. Available at: file:///C:/Users/user01/Downloads/GG-POS-2017-Bross.pdf [Accessed: 2025-October-08]

[40] EBM Network. Evidenzbasierte Medizin und Daseinsfürsorge statt erlösgesteuerter Gefährdung des Patientenwohls! [Evidence-based medicine and public welfare instead of revenue-driven endangerment of patient well-being!] 2019, www.ebm-netzwerk.de/de/veroeffentlichungen/stellungnahmen-pressemitteilungen [Accessed: 2025-October-25]

[41] Bundesministerium für Gesundheit (Federal Ministry of Health). Evidenzbasierte Medizin [Evidence-based Medicine] 2025; https://www.bundesgesundheitsministerium.de/ [Accessed: 2025-June-19]

[42] (Zentrale Ethikkommission) bei der Bundesärztekammer [Central Ethics Committee of the German Medical Association]. Ärztliches Handeln zwischen Berufsethos und Ökonomisierung. Das Beispiel der Verträge mit leitenden Klinikärztinnen und -ärzten [Medical practice between professional ethics and economization. The example of contracts with senior hospital physicians]. DtschArztebl. 2013;**110**:38

[43] Thöns M. Patient Ohne Verfügung [Patients without Advance Directives]. München: Piper; 2016

[44] Galle J. Klugentscheiden ... in der Inneren Medizin [Decide wisely ... in internal medicine]. DtschArztebl. 2019;**116**:16

[45] Parsa-Parsi RW. The Revised Declaration of Geneva: A modern-day physician's pledge. JAMA. 2027;**318** (20):1971–1972. DOI: 10.1001/jama.2017.16230

[46] Nida-Rümelin J quoted in Fuhr Ch. Ethik in der Medizin – Gefährdet die Ökonomisierung das ärztliche Berufsethos [Ethics in medicine – Does economization threaten the Medical Profession's ethics?]. Gynäkologie Und Geburtshilfe. 2017, **22**, 43–53

[47] Tagesschau.de Das sind die Eckpunkte der Krankenhausreform [These are the key points of the hospital reform] 2023; https://www.tagesschau.de/inland/innenpolitik/krankenhausreform-110.html [Accessed: 2025-June-02]

[48] InEK -Institut für das Entgeltsystem im Krankenhaus [InEK – Institute for the Hospital Remuneration System]. Erlösvolumen für die Versorgung von Kindern und Jugendlichen [Revenue volume for the care of children and adolescents]; 2024, https://www.g-drg.de/erloesvolumen-fuer-die-versorgung-von-kindern-und-jugendlichen. [Accessed: 2025-October-25]

[49] Fäßler M, Biller-Andorno N. Die Diskussion um Chefarzt-Boni in Deutschland und der Schweiz [The debate surrounding bonuses for chief physicians in Germany and Switzerland]. In: Dieterich A, Braun B, Th G, Simon M, eds. Geld Im Krankenhaus - Eine Kritische Bestandsaufnahme Des DRG-Systems [Money in Hospitals – A Critical Assessment of the DRG System]. Wiesbaden: Springer Fachmedien; 2019. p. 161–186. DOI: 10.1007/978-3-658-24807-9_8

[50] Klundt M. Kinderrechte in Corona-Zeiten [Children's rights in the age of coronavirus]. Stimmen der Zeit. 2021;**146**(1):13–23

[51] Schlögl-Flierl K. Vaccination? Between the right to self-determination and the common good. Stimmen der Zeit. Vaccination. 2021;**146**(1):3–11

[52] Staudt F. Medical Ethics: Epikeia and Proportionality. American Journal of Pediatrics and Neonatology. 2025;**1**(1)

[53] Gilbert A, Ghuysen A. Triage in the time of COVID-19. The Lancet Digital Health. 2022;**4**(4):e210–e211

[54] Miller D, Moss A. Rethinking the ethics of the COVID-19 pandemic lockdowns. Hastings Center Report. 2023;**53**(4):3–9. DOI: 10.1002/hast.1495

[55] Spahn J, Köhne O, Käfferlein P. Wir Werden Einander Viel Verzeihen Müssen: Wie Die Pandemie Uns Verändert Hat – Und Was Sie Uns Für Die Zukunft Lehrt. Innenansichten Einer Krise [We will have to forgive each other a lot: How the Pandemic has changed Us –and What It teaches us for the future. Inside views of a Crisis]. München: Heyne Verlag; 2022

[56] Berndt C, Grill M. Masken-Affäre: Wie Jens Spahn Steuermilliarden versenkte [Mask affair: How Jens Spahn sank billions in tax money]. Süddeutsche Zeitung. 2025-June-06. https://www.sueddeutsche.de/politik/jens-spahn-maskenbeschaffung-regierung-li.3265242?reduced=true [Accessed: 2025-October-25]

[57] Klein N. The Shock Strategy: The Rise of Disaster Capitalism. New York: Metropolitan Books; 2007

[58] Stiftung Dialog Ethik. Ein Eid für heutige Ärztinnen und Ärzte [An oath for today's doctors]. Schweiz Ärztezeitung. 2015;**25**:930–934

[59] Schumm-Draeger PM. Medizin vor Ökonomie – DGIM rückt Wertediskussion in den Fokus [Medicine Before Economics - DGIM is Focusing on Discussion of Values]. Deutsche Medizinische Wochenschrift. 2017;**142**(7):461. DOI: 10.1055/s-0042-121497

[60] Hensold S. 215 Ärzte Fordern: Mensch Vor Profit! [215 Doctors Demand: People before Profit!] *Stern* Ed. 37. 2019; https://www.stern.de/gesundheit/aerzte-appell [Accessed: 2025-October-25]

[61] Imabe. Institut für Medizinische Anthropologie und Bioethik. Deutscher Ärztetag: „Patientenwohl muss ethischer Maßstab für das Krankenhaus sein“ [German Medical Association: “Patient welfare must be the ethical benchmark for hospitals”]. 2026; https://www.imabe.org/bioethikaktuell/einzelansicht/deutscher-aerztetag-patientenwohl-muss-ethischer-massstab-fuer-das-krankenhaus-sein [Accessed: 2025-October-25]

[62] Gutmann Th. Würde und Autonomie. Überlegungen zur Kantischen Tradition [Dignity and Autonomy. Reflections on the Kantian Tradition]. Preprints of the Centre for Advanced Study in Bioethics, Münster 2010; file:///C:/Users/user01/Downloads/02_gutmann_-_w_rde_und_autonomie1.pdf

[63] Maio G. Mittelpunkt Mensch. Ethik in der Medizin. Ein Lehrbuch, 2. Erweiterte Auflage [Focus on People: Ethics in Medicine: A Textbook, 2nd Expanded Edition]. Stuttgart: Schattauer; 2017

[64] Babić J. The Golden Rule and the Categorical Imperative. Ethical Thought. 2022;**22**(1):37–50. DOI: 10.21146/2074-4870-2022-22-1-37-50

[65] Kardinaltugenden SD: Bedeutung einfach erklärt [Cardinal virtues: Meaning explained simply]. Focus Online. 2025-April-27; https://praxistipps.focus.de/kar-dinaltugenden-bedeutung-einfach-erklaert_186995 [Accessed: 2025-October-25]